# Toilet-Training & Bed-Wetting

A common-sense approach, based on parents' experiences

# Toilet-Training & Bed-Wetting

## A PRACTICAL GUIDE FOR TODAY'S PARENTS

*by*

**Heather Welford**

THORSONS PUBLISHING GROUP
Wellingborough, Northamptonshire

First published 1987

© HEATHER WELFORD 1987

*All rights reserved. No part of this book may be reproduced or utilized in any form or by any means, electronic or mechanical, including photocopying, recording or by any information storage and retrieval system, without permission in writing from the Publisher.*

British Library Cataloguing in Publication Data

Welford, Heather
Toilet-training and bed-wetting
1. Bed-wetting
I. Title
649'.62      HQ784.T6

ISBN 0-7225-1344-5

Printed and bound in Great Britain

3  5  7  9  10  8  6  4  2

# CONTENTS

|  | Page |
|---|---|
| *Foreword* | 9 |
| *Introduction — The Physical Basics* | 11 |

**Part One: Toilet Training** — 17
1. What do we mean by toilet training? — 19
2. What do other parents do? — four approaches — 24
3. General principles — 34
4. A suggested programme of training — 38
5. Potties, pants and the naming of parts... — 43
6. Coping with accidents — 48
7. Out and about — visits and holidays during training — 53
8. When all else failed — stories of unexpected success — 58
9. 'Over-night' success — how to get rid of night-time nappies — 60
10. Special situations — twins, the handicapped child — 65

**Part Two: Problems** — 71
11. Delays in achieving bladder and bowel control — 73
12. Physical problems — 80
13. Wetting during the day — 90
14. Bed-wetting — 94
15. Soiling — 112
16. Where to find help — 120
    *Questions and Answers* — 122
    *Index* — 141

# ACKNOWLEDGEMENTS

This book could not have been written without the help of well over 100 parents — mainly mothers. They took the trouble to answer a questionnaire I sent them about their experiences, or else wrote to me in response to my request in *Parents* magazine. In addition, many other mothers have talked to me informally, both during the preparation of this book and also in the years leading up to it, long before Thorsons asked me to consider writing on the topic of toilet-training, when I was researching the subject for magazine articles. My thanks go to all those parents, as I hope their individual and collective experiences will be of great value to everyone reading this book.

I also want to thank the people I have worked with on the *Parents* problem pages, especially Alison Spiro, Juliet Hopkins and Professor Eric Stroud — health visitor, psychotherapist and paediatrician respectively. None of them has been directly concerned with the text of this book, but all of them have, through their experience and sympathetic approach, taught me a great deal about children, and about families.

Clinical psychologist Jennifer Adams gave me valuable help and advice during the research period, and I thank her and health visitor Maggie Murray and senior clinical medical officer Dr A. Carruthers for allowing me the chance to sit in on their clinics, in the West Midlands and in Gateshead, Tyne and Wear.

Dorothy Haywood looked after my youngest child while this book was in preparation. All working mothers will understand when I say I am truly grateful to have had someone so reliable and so caring in this position of trust.

At very short notice, Pauline Rossen typed the final manuscript, and gave a highly valuable mother's-eye-view of the text in its last stages, in time for me to make important amendments and additions.

*Heather Welford*

# FOREWORD

'It's not toilet-*training*, it's toilet-*teaching*!' pleaded a colleague when I asked her to tell me about her experiences. 'Children aren't animals.'

She's right, of course. Learning about bowel and bladder control is a normal part of a child's development that we, as parents, merely help them to achieve. It shouldn't be a problem, and it shouldn't be a question of you imposing your will on your child, as you might do while training an animal in behaviour he wouldn't otherwise naturally do. It's natural for humans to empty bowels and bladder according to certain socially-approved practices. This is the case at all points in history and in all societies. So why is it a problem? Why should a parent want to seek their doctor's, health visitor's, magazine's, neighbour's, friend's advice because it's causing them anxiety? Why do so many parents feel it's gone wrong?

I think the reason is at least partly to do with the way many young mothers and fathers lack confidence. They are thrown in at the deep end of parenthood with the birth of their first child and they have to learn as they go. Previous generations lived more closely together and they had more children — adults starting a family of their own remembered having younger siblings and cousins around, and child rearing wasn't a completely separate part of life. Today, things are very different. There's a lack of family support, and young parents may find it difficult to make new contacts to replace this. They may not know what to do or where to start.

This book will answer some of the worries that arise when lack of information and lack of confidence combine

— but it will not tell you exactly how to toilet-train. That is for you to decide, on the basis of what you feel is right for you and your child. I don't feel anyone can dictate 'methods' of parenting, and that goes for all areas of family life.

I do believe, though, that other parents' experiences are both interesting and informative, and that's why I have included many real-life accounts, case histories, problems and solutions. The work done by doctors and therapists in the area of training is valuable too, and I have aimed to find up-to-date, relevant and helpful research studies. This is especially the case in Part Two which deals with the difficulties, both physical and emotional, that can affect children — and affect them at times very profoundly. Bed-wetting is a major part of this section, as it should be, because it's a very common problem and one which can cause quite extensive frustrations for the child involved and her family.

If you have any stories to share about your own experiences, please let me know of them. I would find them useful for future editions of this book.

*Heather Welford*

## Author's note

I haven't followed the usual practice of calling children 'he' in this book. Here — in line with real life — a child is sometimes 'he' and sometimes 'she', and sometimes 'he or she'.

# INTRODUCTION — THE PHYSICAL BASICS

All healthy humans share the same basic physical functions, whether they're adults or children, though the finer details of the way the functions work may take time to develop through infancy, childhood and adolescence. Some, like the reproductive system, lie ready but waiting for some years.

We have physical functions that work totally outside our conscious control, such as the circulation of the blood. Other functions depend on us to make an act of will to stimulate them — the movements of our limbs fall into this category. Still other body actions, like breathing, can be brought under a limited measure of control if we want to. The digestive system, and the way our bodies get rid of waste products, have elements of all three categories. Eating and drinking are voluntary activities, though they may be prompted by the involuntary stimuli of hunger and thirst; the way the digestive tract works on the food or drink is beyond our control; when and where we eliminate the waste is to a great extent dependent on a conscious decision, though the urge that prompts us is usually involuntary.

In most societies, the *when* and especially the *where* of elimination, at least as far as adults and children beyond infancy are concerned, is highly controlled. We're concerned that the act is private and solitary, that it happens in a particular place, and we usually expect to wait until an appropriate time to do it (disappearing in the middle of a meal or a conversation is usually considered not the correct moment). Being able to obey all these norms is something we learn as a child.

It's not the purpose of this book to examine why we have these standards of behaviour, or particularly to question them. I'm starting off by simply accepting the fact that for our children, adopting these norms is a way of becoming acceptable to others in all social situations. When children over a certain age (variable as that may be, as we'll see) for whatever reason don't conform to these norms, it's regarded as a problem. Parents often want to know how they can lead their sons and daughters to the stage of conforming — to the stage of being 'trained' — and avoid problems developing.

It's interesting to look at the way the bowels and bladder work in adult human beings, and to compare that with the way they operate in babies and children. (For simplicity's sake, I won't use this section to deal wth the way non-physical factors can exert an influence on physical functioning, as these areas will be covered elsewhere in the book.)

## The Bladder

The adult bladder can hold about 280ml (half a pint) of urine before the urge to urinate — to get rid of it — is felt. The kidneys are where urine is made, as a result of their function of regulating the water and salt contents of the blood. The kidneys are working all the time to dispose of excess fluid and unwanted waste matter to maintain the right balance. Both kidneys are made up of a collection of very fine tubes called nephrons, each one of which leads to one of the two ureters, large tubes leading in turn to the bladder. The nephrons have the job of absorbing salts, sugars and other nutrients from the blood and filtering out what isn't wanted as urine, which passes into the ureters. From there, muscle contractions push the urine into the bladder at the rate of several bursts of urine each minute.

The bladder wall is made up of muscular tissue, and it allows itself to stretch as it fills, rather like a balloon. When the muscles are stretched beyond a certain point, the pressure triggers off a reflex contraction which your brain interprets as the need to pass urine. At the exit point of the bladder is a ring of muscle — called a sphincter muscle —

that normally keeps the bladder closed. When you want to open the bladder to allow the urine to flow, you can voluntarily relax the muscle. The urine then passes through the urethra, which is a small canal, leading from the bladder to the vulva (in women) and to the penis (in men). The average adult needs to pass urine something like half a dozen times a day, and the total passed is about one and a half litres (three pints).

In a small baby, the physiology of urination is similar, though the kidneys are comparatively immature in their functioning, and aren't designed to cope with a high salt intake or to withstand dehydration. Urine is stored in the bladder in much the same way as in the adult, though the capacity of the bladder starts off very small, and grows throughout infancy and childhood. Once a newborn is feeding frequently, the bladder empties a stream of urine up to 20 times a day. In one study of breastfed infants, the amount passed averaged about 200 ml (approximately a third of a pint) on the 10th day after birth[1]. Another study tabulated the increase in volume of urine through childhood, and demonstrated the way it doubles between the ages of one year and eight years and doubles again between eight and fourteen[2].

In a baby, the emptying of the bladder is a totally involuntary action, and the sphincter opens in response to the fullness of the bladder, though the reflex can be conditioned to respond to other stimulation like the rim of the potty being placed on the baby's bottom (see page 26). The frequency of emptying seems to decrease as the months go on, and parents will notice that as their baby grows, her nappy is less likely to be wet every time it's felt.

At some point over the next three years or so, the child becomes aware that she's passed urine. Some babies, it's true, seem to know when their nappies are wet, though they don't have any idea that they are responsible for the wetness. In my experience the baby who's bothered about wetness is the exception — more often, he's unruffled and apparently ignorant of a soaking, even leaking, nappy unless there is some discomfort or pain from a nappy rash or urine infection.

The next stage is when the child knows she's going to pass urine in the next second or so. This feeling is known as 'urgency'. Then, as the child learns to recognize and respond to the signs that her bladder needs emptying, the urgency becomes less acute. The child can 'hang on' more and more, not just by contracting her pelvic-floor muscles to close off the urethra but by deliberately controlling the sphincter muscle by not releasing it. This ability to hang on increases with general physical and social maturity, and with the growing capacity of the bladder. Later, she can also release the sphincter without having felt the need to urinate.

## The Bowel

The function of the bowel in human beings is to complete the digestion and absorption of food begun earlier in the digestive tract, and to send waste material to the rectum where it is stored and later excreted as faeces. The colon (or large bowel, called thus to make a distinction between it and the small bowel) is what the lay person means when he refers to the 'bowel'. It is a muscular tube, which would measure about 1.5 metres (five feet) in length if it were uncoiled. It re-absorbs much of the water in the waste matter that arrives there, and forms the semi-solid faecal mass (or motion or stool). The rectum distends when it is full of faeces and this produces the urge to defecate or 'open the bowels'.

The faeces emerge through the anus, which is the small channel that opens between the buttocks. Like the bladder there is a ring of muscle closing the anus — the anal sphincter — and it's the voluntary relaxing and contracting of the sphincter and 'pushing', by exerting pressure within the abdomen, that allows the faeces to be pushed out. In a healthy person, the bowel motion is fairly soft and it is passed without any difficulty. Frequency varies — about once or twice a day is average.

The baby's first bowel motion is called meconium — it's very sticky and it's passed within the first day or so after birth. It's formed mainly of mucus, dead cells and amniotic fluid. Over the next few days the stools change, and if the

## INTRODUCTION—THE PHYSICAL BASICS

baby is feeding normally, by a week or so they will be very loose and daffodil-yellow (if breastfed) or pale brown and firmer (if fed on baby formula). Formula-fed babies pass stools fairly regularly. Breastfed babies are less predictable. Half-a-dozen stools a day — or more — is normal, as is going several days between stools.

Mothers often notice that the bowels of a new baby move as soon as he starts to feed — the action of feeding and swallowing sets off the reflex which opens the anal sphincter. It can be quite some time before a child becomes aware of having passed a motion (although some babies dislike being in a dirty nappy, they don't know why it feels like that). Again on the pattern of bladder control, the knowledge that she's about to pass a motion is the next stage reached by the child — and from there she gets to the point where the urge to defecate is not too urgent to prevent getting to a pot or lavatory in time.

Under normal circumstances, faeces are only passed when there is a feeling of need to respond to a full rectum, so it's not exactly parallel to bladder control in this respect. We don't usually get quite to the point of being able to defecate at will, though the bowel can be trained to respond to certain stimuli. This can be important when for some reason children fail to recognize the need to pass a motion (see Chapter 15).

Once beyond babyhood, most children on a normal diet pass a stool once or twice a day. Less frequently than this is also normal, as long as the stool is not hard or difficult to pass.

1. D.G. Vulliamy (1982 edition) *The New Born Child* (Churchill Livingstone)
2. G.H. Lowrey (1973 edition) *Growth and Development of Children* (Yearbook Medical Publishers Inc)

# PART ONE: TOILET-TRAINING

# 1.

# WHAT DO WE MEAN BY TOILET-TRAINING?

Bladder and bowel control are actually the final stage in a sequence of developments. The ability to reach that stage depends on physical *and* emotional maturity. The knowledge of where to put the urine and the faeces has to be passed on and accepted. That is, we need to tell our children that the place and time to open the bowels and the bladder is the potty or the lavatory, when it's the right time to respond, and our children have to understand and act on that. However, children observe and copy others in many other areas of life without specific instructions or constant reminders. Is there any need for an active role on the part of an adult, to instigate and continue a process the child will engage in anyway?

In fact, we will be looking at the option of not actively 'training' at all, and just leaving your child to make his own progress (see page 26). However, when we examine what most parents actually decide to do in our society, and how children respond, it's clear that the majority of families have some sort of positive programme involving the steps taken between the stage of nappies all the time and final independence — even if the programme, as such, is very relaxed. Few leave it completely up to the child, though attitudes, expectations and practices have become less interventionist over recent years.

**When are most children trained?**
We know the age range within which most children start walking (between 10 months and 18 months), the average age for the first word (about 12 months), and many other important milestones, as they're called, are well-

documented. Similar sorts of statistics should give us an idea of what we could call reasonable expectations when it comes to learning about bowel and bladder independence. But it's not as easy as that. Whereas expectations of such attainments as sitting, walking and talking remain within the same age ranges across the years, this is not true of bowel and bladder control. For example, one of this country's leading paediatricians, and a writer of many standard works on child health and development, states the age of 18 months as the point at which the normal child is 'clean and dry with only (the) occasional accident'.[1] My own observations and the experience of the mothers in my survey (see acknowledgements) suggests that this is an unusually early age. Most children of this age are still in nappies. The first edition of that book was published in 1953 and I would guess that the 18-month-old clean and dry toddler would be the result of some fairly extensive and intensive training commencing most likely some time before the first birthday. Another popular baby care book published in the 1950s urges mothers strongly *not* to give training a thought until after the first year — negative encouragement of this kind in baby books is always a sure sign of what mothers are actually doing at the time — though it allows the idea of regular potting if the baby is willing[2]. The training would involve a lot of quick work producing potties at exactly the right moment, preceded by varying periods holding even the smallest of babies over the pot, and at 18 months the toddler would still depend on the mother taking much of the initiative in the situation.

When asking mothers about their own families' experiences, I asked them to regard a 'trained child' as one who is able to use the lavatory (or potty) reasonably independently, perhaps with help over clothing and bottom-wiping. Two to two-and-a-half was the commonest age, and it was not unusual for a child to reach this stage well after three without there being any underlying health or emotional problems, or other developmental delay. It's significant that a book first published in 1986 talks about two-and-a-half years being the age at which 'most children can tell their parents by word or gesture that they need to

## WHAT DO WE MEAN BY TOILET-TRAINING?

pass urine and are usually able to hang on for a few minutes'[3].

Night-time training follows a similar pattern over the last generation. Parents 30 years ago might expect night nappies to be discarded at about the age of two, though they may well have continued to 'lift' the child to visit the pot or toilet in order to help ensure a dry bed. My survey indicated that it's not until the third birthday that, in general, parents start to be concerned about night-time.

There are some consistencies across the years, however. It seems clear that on the whole girls are quicker than boys to gain control — this factor is born out by both older and newer text-books, and also by my survey. This applies to the day and night. It's wrong to be dogmatic, of course, as some girls are slower than some boys, and some boys are relatively quick. The text-books also support the notion that bowel control is reached before bladder, though admittedly there are many exceptions to this in my observations.

Interestingly, problems with lack of control, presenting either as bed-wetting or as problems with day-time wetting or soiling, show up as a consistent percentage, too, with no significant change over time (though different countries show different rates — why is a matter for speculation). This would suggest that problems of this sort are unaffected by the way general child care practices change. The percentage of five-year-old children who regularly wet the bed as reported in one text-book[4] was 10 per cent, falling to five per cent at the age of ten, and then to between one and two per cent in the teens. Day-time wetting is considerably lower — about one per cent in the seven to ten-year age group. Problems with soiling affect about one per cent of seven-year-olds. (More detailed statistics about these problems will be found in Part Two).

Although most parents would regard problems such as bed-wetting and soiling over about five or six, as undesirable, there's little doubt that today we have more relaxed ideas about basic training. This isn't just because we have a more child-centred, more liberal approach to family life than we used to — though I wouldn't under-estimate this. The grandmother who wrote to me saying that another grandmother had told her that 'six months, exactly six months, is the age for a baby to make friends with the potty' was expressing a rigidity of approach that is simply out of step with the way most of us bring our children up today. Most parents feel that where individuals are concerned, cast-iron expectations and unbendable rules about when to introduce anything are misplaced. (Not that I'm suggesting for one minute that my own generation of parents has all the answers — far from it! I'm merely reporting what I find current attitudes to be.)

With toilet-training though, practicalities have at least as great a role to play as underlying philosophy. The marketing manager for a brand of disposable nappy who told me (not without pleasure) that mothers were leaving their children in nappies for longer because the industry was making such excellent products was actually speaking sense. More and more babies and toddlers these days are wearing disposable nappies instead of traditional terry-towelling squares, and the increase in their use has a lot to do with the improved fit and performance compared to the lack-lustre, only semi-absorbent disposables of the 1970's. And today's disposables are a miracle compared with the useless oblongs of gauze-covered cotton available in the 60's. The cost of disposables has kept below inflation, so they have become less of a luxury item, too. Even mothers who've stuck with terries find that washing them in an automatic washing-machine (and perhaps drying them in a tumble-dryer) is not that great a headache — at least not compared with the daily boil-up in a copper boiler on the stove that was the usual method only 20 years ago. And then, you had to wring them out and get the things dry. Of course, given woman's resourcefulness, most people managed okay for lack of an alternative, but today it does seem that mums don't mind that much about nappies, now that the hard work's gone out of them. The push to save the occasional nappy by early potty-training is not there any more. It could also be that we are more likely to leave it all until later, when success comes more quickly, than risk the inevitable oceans of puddles and mess on the Axminster.

When houses weren't carpeted wall-to-wall throughout, their floors were easier to wipe clean!

1. R.S. Illingworth (1983 edition) *The Normal Child* (Churchill Livingstone)
2. Ruth Martin *Before the Baby and After* (Hurst and Blackett, 1958)
3. D. Hull *The Macmillan Guide to Child Health* (Guild Publishing, 1985)
4. P. Barker *Basic Child Psychiatry* (Collins, 1983)

# 2.

# WHAT DO OTHER PARENTS DO? — FOUR APPROACHES

This chapter will contain details of four different approaches to bowel and bladder control. I hesitate to use the word 'method' though, as you'll see, you can be very methodical if you wish, by making one stage lead on to another, and some approaches need a definite consistency and commitment on the part of the adult involved.

If you've already had a go at potty-training and have abandoned the whole idea in anger or despair (or both), then starting again with these suggestions in mind may be all you and your child need. If you've decided to leave actual training to your child and nothing has happened to show that progress is being made, you may decide to step in and move things along with an idea culled from the next few pages. If you think you and your child are ready but you don't have much idea of the best way to go about it, reading these sections may also help.

None of the following approaches needs to be regarded as infallible. Even the Intensive Approach (page 28) doesn't have to be followed slavishly. No book can give you any more than adaptable guidelines for you to mould, reject, re-adopt and then change as you see fit, bearing in mind your home circumstances, your temperament and your child's needs. I've based the information on what mothers have told me, and everything that's suggested comes from real life and practical experience — but of course it may not be appropriate for your child.

## 1. The Early Approach

'I'd intended starting to potty-train early but I hadn't thought I would do it quite as soon as I did — it's just the way it worked out. I always changed Laura's nappy after a feed, but I found she wet it almost straight away every time. So when she was three months old I started sitting her on her potty after each feed. I was a bit unsure of the idea, and I had no way of knowing what Laura would think of it, but she was quite happy. In fact, she giggled! I used a very small potty until she was nine months old, and until she could sit up I obviously had to hold her. Within a week or so of starting, she seemed to get the idea and she was passing water about half the time, and she started opening her bowels in it too. When she was 8 months, she was going up to five days with wet nappies only — I was managing to catch each of her motions, during this time. She started saying "good girl" at about this age, too, which is what I always said to praise her. I began looking at books with her when she was using the potty and she was never unhappy about sitting there. At between 10 and 12 months old she became clean, as she was able to let me know when she wanted to have a poo, and although she was still in nappies at a year, they were usually dry. I was putting her on the potty between seven and nine times a day. She began asking for her potty at 16 months, and by 18 months she was asking most of the time, with only the occasional accident; at 20 months she started wearing ordinary pants instead of the trainer pants she'd been wearing for the last month or so at home. When I took her out, though, I still took a potty if I was going anywhere without a toilet, and I usually took spare pants too, "just in case". Not long afterwards, she was able to be trusted in ordinary pants all day, wherever we went. She's almost 3 now, and uses the toilet most of the time, though she needs help to get on as she's on the small side.'

*Jenny*

Jenny's approach, as we saw on page 22, is unusual in these days of disposable nappies and automatic washing machines. Laura was clean and dry in most situations some time before the age of two, and certainly that's sooner than most children, though not dramatically so.

In fact, babies can be *conditioned* to use the potty at a very young age. The bladder and bowel reflex actions come into play as a response to the feel of the potty. However, this is different from conscious control. Early success in this form of training often comes to an end when the baby gets to be a toddler and starts being able to control the reflex.

'Six months was far too soon to start potting. It became a struggle and he was three before I would say he was fully trained. Training was much easier with my next child, after I left it later.'
*Paula*

With Laura, the transition between reflex actions and voluntarily control was very smooth — perhaps because of a placid temperament or because her mother was happy never to force the issue. Jenny potted Laura seven to nine times a day — that's about once every waking hour if Laura still had a daytime nap. If that sounds to you like hard work — well, it does to me as well! But it might well suit you if you only have one child, or if your baby has much older, less demanding siblings, and you don't have an especially busy life — or if you just like the idea of saving the odd nappy, and giving your baby the chance to have a sense of achievement in this way.

Jenny's calm and unpressurizing attitude was, I feel, crucial in keeping the whole potty scene happy and rewarding. It sounds as if Laura had plenty of accidents in between the dry nappies in the 15 months or so (whew!) her mother was actively training her, so Jenny needed to stay unambitious. Jenny obviously felt it was worth it, but not everyone would feel that way, or remain patient for over a year of training.

## 2. The Child's Initiative Approach

'My children are now aged six years and four years. I left the decision of when to train up to them — in fact, neither of them were really "trained" in the ordinary sense. They both made the choice to stop wearing nappies at the age of $2\frac{1}{4}$. Because Bobby, the eldest, had done it so successfully, I

had never taken the initiative with Lee, his younger brother. I was quite happy to wait. In some ways it was easy when he was in nappies, as I'm a keep-fit teacher and I was taking Lee to class with me, so he had no extensive time at home where we could have concentrated on training. As it turned out, the half-term break came along when he decided he didn't want nappies any more, and of course I let him know of my encouragement and support. There were a few accidents, but only for a few days — and we both took them in our stride. The change from nappies to pants was a non-event.'
*Lin*


'Susie had a try of the potty at about 20 months on my suggestion but I quickly abandoned the idea as she wouldn't sit still on it, and the subject hardly came up again. Then one evening when she was $2\frac{1}{2}$, she opened her bowels in the bath — I didn't get cross, but just pointed out that she could ask me for the potty next time. She asked for it there and then, and produced another poo quite happily. The next morning I put a pretty pair of knickers on her instead of a nappy, explaining what I expected of her. She started straight away, using the potty of her own accord without any prompting, and managed her clothing very well. After a short while she started using the toilet instead. I had always felt rather lacking when other toddlers were using the potty at 18 months or so and Susie was not, but now in retrospect I think I was right to leave it until she felt herself that she was good and ready'.
*Fiona*


'When Tina was 25 months exactly, I was dressing her in the morning and she said the magic words "no nappy". She had shown no previous interest in the idea of doing without nappies, though we had asked if she'd like to try. That morning she just wore pants, and after a few days of accidents she has been clean and dry both day and night.'
*Maggie*

Generally, leaving it up to your child to let you know when she wants to go without nappies will mean waiting until after the second birthday. (This is not always the case — one of the mums in the survey responded to the clear desire of her 14-month-old son to use the potty. She would not have thought of actively training as soon as this.) This might be too long if you are keen to move your child on to independence and control sooner than this, and on the whole it probably means a longer period in nappies. However, the advantage is that the child seems to know pretty accurately how capable she is and there is only a very short period of puddles and mess before full control. There is no risk of adult impatience with a child who's just not ready to go without nappies, and the child is always pleased, not resentful, at your encouragement. It helps greatly if the child has had the chance to know what potties and toilets are for, and to have gained awareness of her bowel and bladder productions.

Tina's mum, Maggie, had further thoughts: 'I have seen many two-year-olds who have never been taught to be aware of their bodily functions — then they're suddenly expected to control them. As soon as a child starts walking, she can have a chance to go without a nappy for an unaccustomed sense of freedom and the chance to do a pee or a poo without a nappy on — you can have a pot close at hand if you want.'

## 3. The Intensive Approach

'I've done this twice, with both my sons. It took a couple of days each time — certainly no more. With the younger one it was really quick as the older boy helped him. He was about $2\frac{3}{4}$ and I just decided "today is the day". I got a pile of old shorts and pants handy, together with the potty and just told him "when you need a wee, do it in the pot". With help he got the hang of it in a single morning. I gave him loads to drink — orange squash — so he'd need to go often, and which helped to train the bladder. When it came to going out that same day I got him to wee before we went, then when we came back. We abandoned the potty after the first two or three days and the loo was used instead. I

deliberately adopted a very relaxed attitude as I'd seen loads of friends get neurotic about wet clothes, wet beds, wet sheets, wet car seats and wet parents — no-one seemed to have the courage to leave off training because of pressure from other people and some worry that their children were behind in some way.'
*Delia*


'I was walking through a bookshop one afternoon and a book title caught my eye. It was *Toilet Training in Less than a Day*[1]. I'd been thinking about potty-training Caroline, and I bought it. It describes a method of toilet-training that the authors virtually guarantee will work if it's followed meticulously with a child who's ready for training anyway. I tried it, and it worked really well; Caroline was dry at night after it too, at only 22 months. I used the same method again with my second daughter two years later. She was the same age as Caroline had been. It didn't work quite so well, as we couldn't stay in all day and I couldn't give Isobel full attention all the time with Caroline around. However it was still a quick way to train — it only took a few days.'
*Pam*


Taking the initiative in this way and deciding firmly and confidently that your child can and will be trained can be very successful if you pick the right moment. The book mentioned by Pam (see notes) is worth reading if you can find a copy (it's out of print) as it contains much common sense, even if you don't follow every point of its instruction. Some suggestions are the same as those implemented by Delia — plenty to drink, and plenty of spare pants for insurance. You do need to set aside a day with no other distractions so you and your child can concentrate on dry pants and the potty. Rewards for dry pants are suggested to re-inforce the message, and the child is encouraged to pull his own pants up and down and to empty the pot into the loo. The authors recommend buying a special wetting doll to demonstrate the use of the potty and to act as a model for the child.

Confidence in the child, and friendly firmness in your own approach is essential, and you do need to be sure your child is ready to understand and follow instructions. Delia's son, at $2\frac{3}{4}$, was certainly old enough to have the language and the ability to co-operate with his mother's plans, but not all 22-month-olds would be as successful at getting the message and acting on it as Pam's daughter Caroline. This intensive approach actually incorporates many of the General Principles outlined in Chapter 3, but it does demand a commitment from you to set aside at least a day and to keep it entertaining. This can be hard work. Sally told me: 'I used the "train in a day" method, and it seemed to work. It wasn't as straightforward as the book suggested, though. I remember Penny (at just turned two) got very bored with "potty talk". It did give her the basic idea, though. Her ability to hang on came later — I spent a lot of time holding her over drains when we went out in the meantime'.

The basic principle behind intensive methods is to create the opportunity for the child to recognize and respond to the signs of a full bladder within a very short time. Actual bladder capacity and more than momentary control will come with physical maturity which may vary between children. When the method works, it can be a very good way of avoiding a long drawn-out training period which *can* lead to frustrations and resentments on both sides.

## 4. Standard British Dead-Slow-and-Stop Approach

'I thought Tom had bladder control when he woke up in the morning with a dry nappy a few times, when he was almost two. I introduced the potty and he began to wear trainer pants in the house, and ran around the garden without any pants on. He pee'd all over the place. I got cross and frustrated, so I put him back into nappies. Two weeks later I tried again, and as long as I made sure he used the potty often enough it worked most of the time. Bowel training was helped by the fact that he had a very regular "after breakfast" habit. I'd sit him on the pot with some drawing paper and crayons and he'd sit there quite happily until he'd finished.'

*Mary*

## WHAT DO OTHER PARENTS DO?—FOUR APPROACHES 31

'I spent a week chasing around with a potty and asking my 20 month-old daughter whether she wanted a wee or a poo and whether she wanted to be a big girl like so-and-so and anything else I felt would entice her to use it. The responses were mainly negative. Then we went on holiday and I gave up the idea and she went back into nappies all the time. We tried again when she was two, and she was almost completely reliable after a week. With my younger child things were different. Emma had seen Nicola use the pot and at 18 months decided she wanted to sit on it too. I thought she seemed to have a bit of control and I took her out of nappies. In retrospect I shouldn't have done. There were frequent accidents and she always needed a nappy if we were going on a car journey of any length or were away from easy access to a loo for more than an hour.'  *Beryl*

'We had a little bit of a problem with bowel control at first, but it resolved itself after three months or so, and although he's almost three now and has been reasonably reliable for six months, he still has periods when he wets his pants and needs reminding to "go".  *Marion*

'Holly was 22 months when I began potty-training. She made good progress in the first week and then things slowed down. We had occasional days without any success at all. Bowel control became a problem. She would say she didn't want to go and then she'd do it in her pants.'
*Barbara*

'Daisy had a rash on her bottom when she was 25 months, and I decided to let her go without a nappy to help clear it up, and to combine that with an attempt at potty-training. That was five months ago, and things have gone very slowly, she still has bowel accidents weekly, though they were daily for the first month or so. A week ago I was saying we now had three bladder accidents a week instead of three (at least!) a day, which it was for about three months. However we've been away for a couple of days and that's put the clock back three or four weeks. Since the

hot weather she's quite often confused the garden with the potty, and over the last 10 days we've had three bowel accidents (though I'm not sure how accidental they were!). I bought a seat and step for the loo about a month into the ordeal, but the novelty soon wore off. I've tried Smarties as a bribe but I don't do it any more as I don't want her to think she can manipulate me. I'm not looking forward to potty-training my next child...'
*Anne*

'It took about 10 days for Judy at 21 months to understand what the potty was for. Once she got the idea, she used it most of the time. Then after two or three months she started wetting her pants, up to six times a day. The doctor checked there was no infection. Bribes or smacks didn't affect it, and it took a whole year before she was reliable again.'
*Angela*

'We introduced the potty when Katie was only 14 months — it was rather soon — and the successes we had at first were accidental. She was clean from 18 months but we'd made no progress whatsoever with wetting. But we went on holiday for a fortnight when she was 26 months and during all that time she was completely clean and dry (day and night). Once we got home, everything went back to normal — that is, she started wetting again. It got worse, as she started soiling as well. She went back into nappies until she was 28 months'.
*John*

(To read what made the difference, see page 58).

I could fill the whole book with case histories like these — training is a long slowish haul up (and sometimes back down) a rather boring hill. This is more or less how parents these days embark on it, and it always works in the end, either because of or in spite of, the parents' persistence. As long as potty-training isn't allowed to become a cause of continual stress because of the slow progress (if any) that's being made, then the only disadvantage of the approach is that it tends to take several months. However, the point about this way of doing things is that the frequent accidents and regressions are frustrating for everyone, occasionally upsetting, and often make a parent angry.

Nevertheless, if you can keep your cool throughout and resist putting training at the top of your list of moans, then this approach could suit you. There's always the chance that training will be quick and easy, if you happen to be lucky.

1. Drs. N. Azrin and R. Foxx
   *Toilet Training in Less than a Day* (Pan, 1977).

# 3.

# GENERAL PRINCIPLES

If, like most parents these days, you don't intend to start any active training until you feel your child's ready, and there's therefore some chance of reasonably quick success, then the following general principles will help you. They aren't rigid — your own child may inspire you to all sorts of creative deviations from your carefully thought-out plan, anyway. And your own circumstances will dictate some of your organization and timing — spending the Christmas holidays with Granny and her expensive pale-coloured carpets is not a good time to start, for example. Nor is it the time when you have the plumbers and builders in to re-do your bathroom and loo facilities.

Having said that, use common sense about ignoring other strictures. I've read articles advising mothers not to start training when they're pregnant (too stressful) or when there's a new baby in the house (not enough time and attention). Obeying both those would account for a whole year of lost time — and given that most women produce their second child between two and four years after the first it's a bit unrealistic. If you do end up, like a lot of us, training during pregnancy or shortly after the birth of a new sibling, see principle number 6.

1. **Talk to your child,** from infancy, about his nappies and the state of them (see Maggie's comments on page 28) — approvingly or matter-of-factly, not critically, if you can help it. Discourage older children from making exaggerated 'Yuk!!' noises at the sight of a dirty nappy.

2. **Don't exclude your baby and toddler from the loo when you use it** — impossible to do this with most children anyway, who will go through phases, varying in length, of wanting to be with you *all* the time. Tell him what you're doing.

3. **Make sure you're reasonably confident of your child's readiness to be trained.** There's no rigid age rule about this. It can happen as early as a year (very rare) or as late as three (not quite so rare). *Most* children don't reach true readiness before 20 months at the very earliest, and the nearer you get to the second birthday the more likely it is that they really are ready. You may have to wait until after this time.

4. **Readiness is physical.** Does your child manage to go for a reasonable time without passing water? This can be difficult to ascertain, especially with today's highly absorbent disposable nappies that simply don't feel wet after only one urination. (There are, however, a couple of brands of disposable now available with a 'wetness-indicator.' A printed design on the outside of the nappy fades and disappears as the nappy dampens.) You may have to leave the nappy off for a short while (on the beach or in the garden makes it easier) and simply observe. What's a 'reasonable' time? Personally, I would feel that a child who needed to urinate more often than every hour and a half or two hours was going to give me a lot of running around and I would feel that was unreasonable. This is particularly the case at the early stages of training when the novelty of it all and the delightful sight of you acting like greased lightning at the request for a potty can combine to make a child 'need' to open her bowels or bladder very often — and I mean *very* often. However, you may be happy about a shorter interval, especially if your child seems keen to learn.

The other physical aspect is co-ordination. Very young children, and others who are just naturally a bit behind in this area, are going to find it difficult to sit comfortably on a potty or toilet, let alone manage to pull pants up and down efficiently. An un-coordinated child may well kick the full potty over as he stands up or catch it with the back of his pants as he struggles to pull them up. That doesn't matter in itself, of course, but it's annoying for you and frustrating for him. You may well prefer to wait until your child can manage to sit on the loo, even if he needs your help in getting on and off (though see the suggestions on page 45).

5. **Readiness is verbal.** Does your child understand simple instructions ('put the cup on the table', 'pick the ball up and give it to daddy')? If not, she's not going to find it easy to understand what you want her to do when she needs to open her bowels or bladder. Her own language ability is less important.

6. **Readiness is emotional.** Is your child going through a reasonably co-operative phase? Toddlers can be extremely negative, they're exploring the effect they have on the world and the people around them — it really is a normal stage and one you just have to learn to cope with in most cases. However, there may be times when your child is rather less negative, and is happy to comply with suggestions from you. Most parents of toddlers learn to manipulate to a certain degree, to exploit their suggestibility and to use their ability to be distracted, so a manageable amount of negative behaviour needn't be an obstacle. After all, you are the boss and you can't let your toddler dictate everything to you! What you do want to avoid is introducing the idea of toilet-training when you're trying to stop your child being say, horribly aggressive with other children, or if he's having a lot of temper tantrums.

Emotional factors may also prevent easy training if your child is going through a major upheaval in his life. This would include divorce or separation between his parents, the recent birth of a new baby (within the previous few weeks) or if he's experiencing some difficulty coping with jealousy of a sibling or other person claiming his mother's attention. Other stressful factors that might interfere with his ability to master the new skill of control could include starting at a day nursery or playgroup; starting with a childminder; a recent stay in hospital (yours or his); a house-move; loss — by death or separation — of someone close to him.

Having said that, you are the one who knows your child best and can gauge the effect that any particular stress or strain has had on him. For example, a stay in hospital may have been for a couple of nights' observation only, throughout which you were able to stay with him, and none of which was painful. Some children will be able to take that in their stride without any distress. However, the same sort of hospital stay can be deeply upsetting to another child, needing time and reassurance to cope with. Making even the gentlest demands to conform to bowel and bladder control on such a child is liable to compound the distress and be unsuccessful. If you attempt training and find your child doesn't seem able to co-operate in some way, and yet you feel he has the physical and verbal readiness outlined above, then it's worth considering if emotional factors are inhibiting him.

7. **Have confidence in your ability to judge the right time,** and in the rightness of your decision. Don't start to train under pressure from other people if you feel it's really not appropriate for you and your child.

'I had never even considered toilet-training Stephen, and then my parents visited when he was 20 months old, and I was 8 months pregnant with my second child. They were *horrified* that he was still in nappies. I followed their advice, though Stephen was entirely unready for it. It caused a lot of unnecessary upset between him and me and he was nearly three when it finally "clicked".   *Jo*

8. **Don't start to train if** you feel you're not up to facing possible set-backs without feeling undermined or angry at your child.

# 4.

# A SUGGESTED PROGRAMME OF TRAINING

If, after reading all these points, you feel you'd like to start training your child, and you feel your child will be willing, you might now wonder how you actually go about it. I hope I've convinced you with what I've already said that there's no one method that is 'the right one'. No two parents train their children in the same way, and there are many individual variations on the theme. However, I've heard from many parents over the years who'd like to be given some definite instructions! Perhaps a mother has found the whole process difficult and unpleasantly frustrating with a previous child, or too long and boring. Or perhaps she has no experience of mixing with other young families and has no one to ask about toilet training. Or perhaps the people she has asked have been the dogmatic type who feel that what they did must be right for everyone... and she doesn't share their outlook.

If you fit into one or more of these categories, or if you just frankly admit that you haven't a clue where to begin, then here's a suggested programme of training. No, I don't think it's necessarily right in every way for your child. And I don't think you should feel you have to follow it point by point. But it is a happy natural sequence of progression that reflects the abilities and understanding of a small child, and builds on success rather than relying on fear of failure. As a generalization the older your child is the quicker he is likely to work through the sequence.

Change the timing of the sequence if you wish, introduce your own tailor-made strategies at each and any point. Abandon the whole thing for another six months! Try something completely different. The programme is yours to

## A SUGGESTED PROGRAMME FOR TRAINING

use as you wish. Do bear in mind that the time span between each point is flexible. Some points may follow more or less immediately after the previous one. Others may be days, weeks or months apart.

1. Buy a potty (see page 43) and put it in the bathroom.
2. Decide on the terminology you'll use (see page 46), and tell your child what the potty is for. ('This for when you want to do a wee/a poo. Big children don't do it in their nappies — they wear pants and use a potty like this, or the loo').
3. Suggest to your child that she sits on it to see what it's like — this can be done with clothes or without, and frequently if she likes the idea.
4. Make a sit-on-the-pot part of your morning routine when dressing your child, and in the evening too, at bedtime.
5. If your child has a regular time for passing a bowel motion (for example, after breakfast or lunch) try and 'catch' the motion by sitting your child on the pot at this time.
6. If and when you catch urine or a stool show pleasure and approval. (Don't go overboard with ecstatic cries of delight).
7. Depending on the willingness of your child, increase the frequency of pot sessions. Look at books with her while she sits on it; if she enjoys watching children's programmes on TV, sit her on the pot while she does so. The point about this increased length of time is that you increase the chances of something ending up in the potty. Never force her to sit on it longer than she wants — many children will never want to sit on it for longer than a few seconds. That's fine.
8. At this stage you can have sessions without pants or nappy on. (If you're training in the summer, and especially if you have a garden, your child may well be used to the freedom of going partially or fully unclothed.) In the morning before getting dressed is sometimes a good time, though it's better if you're around to supervise and produce the potty if you

think it's needed (some households are simply too frantic in the morning for this).

9. Encourage your child to let you know when she has urinated or passed a bowel motion — she will probably be more aware of the bowel motion at first, and may already have reached the stage of letting you know some weeks or even months previously. You can pass on the message about letting you know when you change her. Just say matter-of-factly — 'oh, you're wet. Perhaps you can tell mummy next time and I'll be able to change you nice and quick'. This awareness of *having* urinated or defecated is important and comes before the awareness of an *impending* urination or motion.

10. If you feel you're making good progress, and your child's still happy about the potty, you can step-up the number of times she needs to urinate by increasing the fluid intake. Many children like fruit-flavoured drinks, and they stimulate the kidneys into action more quickly. If your child drinks lemon or orange juice more often than she would normally, you'll be able to re-inforce the potty message more frequently. If you're training more intensively and intend to use rewards, you can give a drink after a successful use of the potty, (see page 58).

11. At some point you're going to have to abandon the use of nappies, at least for your child's waking periods. There is a risk of soiled pants and puddles of course, but you have to accept that. If everything goes well, they may be fewer than you think. Tell your child in advance that you feel sure she'll be able to wear pants instead of nappies — and that in a short while (even tomorrow) you'll buy him/her some big boy's/girl's pants.

12. After showing the pants you've bought, put them on your child instead of a nappy. Older or more dextrous children will be able to put them on themselves and this is certainly something to praise and encourage. It can also make the idea of pants instead of a nappy more attractive, as many (not all) toddlers enjoy feeling independent.

## A SUGGESTED PROGRAMME FOR TRAINING 41

13. Remind your child to ask for the potty if she needs to use it. If you can, put the potty in an accessible place and tell your child where it is. Ideally she should be able to get it and use it without asking/telling you, though this will probably come later.
14. Resist the temptation to ask her to use the potty every 20 minutes (I've seen parents asking as frequently as every 5 minutes). This is boring and irritating for both of you. Frequent reminders may be necessary at times though — for example, if you know she had a long drink of juice an hour ago and is likely to flood the place any second now! Otherwise occasional reminders should be what you aim for.
15. When it comes to going out, encourage your child to use the potty before going — though going before you need to is a skill that's gained later and only older toddlers will be able to oblige straight away. Then put a nappy on (explaining there are no loos on the bus/in the shops etc.) unless you think it's a safe bet she can hang on long enough not to wet her pants (see Chapter 7, *Out and About*, page 53).
16. Continue giving praise and encouragement to your child for using the potty and always respond when he tells you he wants to use it. If you suspect he is asking for the potty more often than he needs, ask yourself whether he likes this way of gaining your attention, or if he's fearful of accidents. If the former, then keep your response more low-key, and if the latter, review your reaction to accidents (see page 48). Either way, move on to the next stage.
17. Encourage greater independence in using the potty. Make sure you have a potty in the room where he's playing (one potty upstairs and one down is helpful) and teach him about pulling clothing up and down and sitting securely on it (little boys need to be told to make sure the penis is pointing down, not out).
18. Introduce him to the idea of using the toilet — and not just your own. He may be happier with a seat (see page 44) and he may well need help in getting on and off if there's no step. Smaller children may need holding on.

19. Throughout, stay happy and unruffled about the whole process. Children quickly learn that 'accidents' can lead to increased attention — don't fall for it! (see Chapter 6, *Coping with Accidents*, page 48).

Again, at the risk of repeating myself, this is no blueprint. I have known no child to follow this programme right the way through in *exactly* this order. It is in fact a simplified synthesis of the way most children can attain control.

# 5.

# POTTIES, PANTS AND THE NAMING OF PARTS

By far the majority of children now use a potty when they are developing bowel control, though their parents certainly expect them to move on to using the lavatory at all times by the time they start school at the very latest.

There are some powerful advantages in using a potty. The main reason is that it's conveniently portable. You can have a potty upstairs and downstairs, you can move it from room to room, and you can grab it and move it to your child when he needs it. All of this is important when your child hasn't yet learnt to hang on for more than a few seconds.

Some parents find it's not too much hassle to take the potty with them on shopping expeditions as well as on visits to potty-less houses, and it can be useful on long car journeys, too (see page 53).

Potties are certainly more comfortable than a toilet to sit on, especially for a younger child, who may be scared of falling down the lavatory bowl, even with a special seat on. Also, it can be easier and more comfortable to pass a bowel motion on the potty — the body is in more of a 'squatting' position, which is, in fact, the correct physiological posture (though our society regards it with distaste).

Potties today are plastic — light, easy to clean and much warmer to sit on than old-fashioned enamel or ceramic types. When choosing one, look for a shape that's stable and easy to lift and carry. Most potties have a 'splash guard' incorporated into the outline, and this is there in the hope (sometimes a vain one) that little boys' urine will stay in the potty rather than be accidentally directed over the edge. Boys should be taught to sit so that the splash guard is at the front, girls should sit with it at the back.

I'm unconvinced of the value of rather more expensive potties designed to look like minature loos, though no doubt someone somewhere has found these the answer to their prayers. I don't feel the extra expense is worth it, and of course they aren't anything like as portable as an ordinary potty. You can buy a chair-shaped potty — in fact it's a chair with its own removable potty rather like a junior commode — with a bar you bring across to stop the child falling off. Again, I remain sceptical. Is it not possible that the child will try to stand up, and then either climb over the bar or topple over it, tipping himself and the potty on to the floor? However, this sort, perhaps with built up sides, is sometimes useful for handicapped children.

Potties shaped like cars or animals are rather jolly, and may help to encourage a child to enjoy sitting there. It's possible that a potty like this could be incorporated into ordinary play more easily, which could endear the child to it even more. However, you'll need to ask yourself if you're prepared to accept the risk that it will be played with when full, or used when it already has a toy in it. Some parents prefer to make the potty's function quite clear-cut from the start.

Think about buying a potty with a lid — not essential, but it does mean you can be discreet about the contents in another person's house or elsewhere when you need to empty it. The lid means that odours are trapped too, which makes carrying and emptying more pleasant. On car journeys, a lidded potty can be kept in the boot if it's been used at the roadside, until you find a place where you can empty it hygienically.

You can keep the potty clean with a rinse-out between uses, and the occasional wash in hot soapy water. Cleaning can be made easier after a bowel motion if you place a piece of toilet paper in the bottom of the potty before your child uses it.

If you've decided to skip the potty stage, or your child seems capable of using the toilet instead, then consider buying a proper child's seat. Many children feel uncomfortable perched on the adult seat, and a tense posture isn't conducive to happy training. A child could be badly frightened by falling into the bowl and even injured. There will be times when the seat won't be around and you may have to hold your child on, or allow her to hold you, but at home a seat can be very helpful. The seats widely available today fit on to most ordinary toilet seats, though your child will probably need help in putting it on correctly. It's a better approach to always have the seat on the loo — older children and adults in the household can remove it when they need to use the lavatory themselves. They should get into the habit of replacing it so it's always ready for the young user.

A small, stable stool or a wooden or plastic box can be placed by the lavatory for the child to use, to help him climb on to the seat. Mothercare produce a 'grow-tall' step, especially for use with the loo or the washbasin, though of course it's got over uses elsewhere too. Another useful product worth investigating is a combined toilet seat and step. This can remian in place when the adult uses the toilet as the seat part is hinged and lifts back.[1]

Trainer pants are thick towelling knickers, with elasticated legs. Most sorts are plastic backed. The idea behind them is that they are worn instead of nappies when a child is not yet reliable — they look like pants, so it's not supposed to be like putting your child in a nappy, but if an accident happens, the urine or motion is contained in the pants and doesn't come through to the clothing. Many parents buy at least a couple of pairs but I have found only a few who found them useful — mainly for outings.

'I use trainer pants when we go out, as Philip (2 years 7 months) is out of nappies in the day, but still has frequent accidents.'
*Chrissie*

More often, they are perceived as actually unhelpful:
'Trainer pants seemed to make things worse. I just took the potty everywhere instead.'
*Una*

'Emily called trainer pants 'nappy pants' and treated them accordingly — she only attempted to control her bowels and bladder in ordinary pants'.

*Sue*

Trainer pants aren't that convenient to wash. They need a hot wash following a dunk in sterilizing solution, just like towelling nappies, and this treatment hardens and cracks the plastic after a time. They also take a very long time to dry. They don't hold as much urine as a nappy, and large deluges flood down the legs.

It seems that trainer pants have very little to offer over putting your child in a nappy, in terms of convenience, though for some children they may give a psychological boost, as a step away from nappies, and perhaps be interpreted as a gesture of trust on your part. I haven't heard of any cases where they made a significant contribution to a child's gain of control — though do let me know if you've found them especially valuable.

It's definitely worth thinking about other clothing for your child, however. Dungarees are of little value when your child needs to get onto a lavatory or potty easily as they can't be unbuckled and pulled down very quickly. It's easiest to keep girls in dresses or in elastic-waisted pull-on trousers or shorts, which is what is best for boys, too. All-in-one snow suits are no good for outdoor wear — ordinary coats or anoraks are better.

What about teaching your child which words to use when talking about his bowel and bladder function? There's a variety of options available, though some of them will leave you absolutely cold, or you'll know straight away you'd find them unacceptable. In fact, sensitive readers should perhaps skip this section!

The English language has a number of 'Anglo Saxon' words that may be considered suitable between close family and friends.

'We'd always wanted to avoid twee baby words with Gareth and we just kept to the words we'd used between ourselves. One day Gareth told his grandparents he wanted "a crap" and they looked so embarrassed. It's no use explaining to a 2½-year-old that some words can be used with mummy and daddy only and he should use other language in front of others. We just had to accept that unless we wanted to make a big thing of using certain words, and not mind about other peoples' feelings we'd have to change our terminology. So it was twee words after all.'

*Jan*


Really, the words you use will depend on what you and your circle find acceptable. Most parents these days use the juvenilisms 'poo' and 'wee' or 'pee', though the other euphemisms 'number one' (for urine) and 'number two' (for a stool) are also used. The Americans have 'B.M.' for bowel motion. Family names — perhaps based on a toddler's mis-pronunciation — sometimes take root and can be passed down the generations! For what it's worth, doctors in the field of working with children with bowel and bladder problems appear to use the words 'poo' and 'wee' when talking directly to parents and children, at least. It's not unreasonable once your child's capable of it, to get him to modify his language in public, especially if his announcements to the world at large are rather loud. You don't need to get him to censor his vocabulary — just to make sure he makes routine requests for the toilet or potty, rather than describing the current urge and what it's for. 'I need the loo, please,' is acceptable in the highest echelons of society (I presume).

1. Eezi-toilet trainer. Details from the manufacturers, Eezi-bath Limited, Unit 8, Mariner, Coton Farm Industrial Estate, Tamworth, Staffordshire B79 7UL. Telephone (0827) 52688.

# 6.

# COPING WITH ACCIDENTS

Unless you're very lucky, or hit exactly the right moment of readiness, your child is going to wet and/or soil his pants. A handful of parents in my survey reported no or virtually no accidents, but by far the majority of these, and other parents I've spoken to, say that wet and dirty pants during the training period, and thereafter, are common.

It's a matter of opinion and judgement whether the accidents are frequent enough to warrant a U-turn on your part. Consider that if your child's not yet able to co-operate — for whatever reason — it might be kinder if you stop reinforcing 'failure' by keeping up requests to use the potty. You can also think about the amount of work involved in mopping up and extra washing that could be saved by a return to nappies. You'll be the best person to guess whether it's worth persevering, taking your child's feelings into account as well as your own. Don't feel it's a step down from your pedestal to bring out the nappies again. Don't feel your child has manipulated you and that he's somehow 'won'. Potty-training should never be regarded as a battleground where you score points off each other in this way.

Let's assume that you've either just started training, or you've decided to continue. Just how do you regard the almost inevitable accident? Rule number one is to regard it as just that — inevitable. Short of strapping a potty to your child's bottom all day, there's no way you can avoid it. Surprise and shock are really out of place. Attitude *is* important and it matters that you're able to commiserate with your child. You can say something like 'Oh, dear. Have you got wet pants? Let's get some dry ones and you can try and use the potty next time'.

## COPING WITH ACCIDENTS

Of course, you might say, that's all very well the first and even the tenth time. What about the tenth time *that day* or the fiftieth time that week? Most parents are, in fact, prepared to remain unaffected by the first few accidents and accidents that are only occasional (however that's defined). It's when they seem to happen more often than expected that attitudes change. I should say here that I'm talking of younger children (particularly the under $3\frac{1}{2}$'s) who have not yet reached reliable day-time dryness or clean-ness. You may want to look at Chapter 11 for a discussion on older children, or ones who have managed to be trained and who have reverted, or who *almost* reached that stage some time ago.

Ways of dealing with repeated accidents vary and parents admit to difficulties:

'Parental patience does not always come easy.' *John*

'I got very cross, smacked him, shut him in the bathroom and consequently deprived him of a lot of love that he desperately needed... it's hard when you've gone through every pair of pants and trousers, especially when everyone else's child picks it up in a month or so and wears the same pair of trousers all day.' *Sonia*

'Frances is two years five months and I'm having a terrible time potty training her... she's always wet, so I just put her in trainer pants plus a nappy pad inside.' *Martine*

'At first I didn't take much notice when Roger wet his trousers. I would just change him without much comment. Now I'm losing my patience and I'm beginning to shout at him. I know I shouldn't, but it makes me really angry.' *Lucy*

It is difficult to keep your temper when you feel your child ought to be able to manage at least a day without wet or dirty pants. Often, mothers suspect their children of deliberately refusing to co-operate, and this makes them even crosser. There may be some truth in this. According to one child psychiatrist writing about bowel control, 'after the first year of life it slowly dawns on a child that what power it has resides in the backside. The child and the child alone chooses whether it will deposit faeces into the potty.... Sometimes through pig-headedness or revenge, it will obstinately withold the little "gifts".[1]

Children develop strategies which can make you quite certain they could do it if they wanted to!

'Paul had such superlative bladder control he found he could relieve the pressure of a full bladder undetected by "leaking" gently, if he was wearing a pair of thick cord trousers. I got cross at this, especially if he was sitting on my knee!'
*Maggie*

Getting wild with rage is really what the child *wants* you to do when this is the case. I know it sounds daft, but sometimes children actually revel in being the focus of your attention, even when that attention is total disapproval. They like you making a fuss. Other children become very anxious as a result of parental anger. It's unhelpful to demonstrate just how important accident-free behaviour is to you. It can actually reinforce the wetting and soiling (see above). And if your child can't help her accidents, it's unkind to be furious with her.

Mothers often report how little positive effect their anger and irritation has on their child's progress — and how unbothered the child is by wet pants.

'I quickly lost count of the number of puddles on the floor when Jodie was being trained, and I was getting madder and madder. One day, after wee'ing yet again, he toddled off to the bathroom, collected the cloth and then proceeded to wipe the floor. Although this brought a smile to my face, I remember thinking "why oh why can't he see the importance of the potty instead of mopping up?"'

*Rita*

Think about it — what does it matter to your child where

## COPING WITH ACCIDENTS

he opens his bowels and bladder? A very young child is miles away from the stage of being bothered what other people think of him, or whether he's acceptable in polite society. He might even like the feel of warm, wet squidgy pants or nappy! Bobby (on page 59) really is an exception. Most children couldn't care less. Sharing that insouciance as far as you are able really can pay dividends.

'I always felt very relaxed about their progress and never tried to compete with other children or mothers — I trusted my own kids' instincts, and looking back I've had far fewer problems that way'.
*Pattie*

If you can't genuinely commiserate with your child (see page 48), no one, least of all me, should dare to suggest you need to be a serene, all-accepting, all-embracing saint of a parent. I don't think it's sensible to pretend that accidents — repeated accidents at that — are just a tiny bit of bad luck if that's not what you feel. The reality of looking after children in today's relatively unsupporting and competitive society means that the pressure can be on you to be top-dog in the potty-trainer stakes. You can even begin to fear your child is retarded or handicapped in some way, and worries about that are difficult to ignore. You may be facing other domestic problems, too, and other aspects of your toddler's apparent stubborness may be getting you down. If you feel angry or extremely 'got at' by floods and messes, and it's hard to keep up with the washing, then accept that's what you feel. You don't need to express those feelings in a show of temper at your child, though. Practise *talking* about your feelings instead of yelling about them or allowing them full rein with a smack. When feeling angry at the umpteenth accident, tell your child, 'Mummy's rather cross at that because she's had to do a lot of washing and wiping-up today. That makes me tired.' Your child has to learn that wet/dirty pants and floors are undesirables — but he doesn't have to feel undesirable or unworthy himself, nor to have the dubious pleasure of knowing just how apoplectic he can make you.

## Practical measures to help you to keep calm.

'I would definitely recommend plastic sandals indoors, instead of shoes and slippers. Slippers in particular are quite revolting when they're soaked in urine (and they disintegrate in the washing machine, or they did when I tried them)...'

*Ruby*


Other tips include keeping up a stock of pants by keeping old ragged ones you'd normally have thrown away in circulation — ditto pyjama trousers for wearing around the house.

It's unrealistic to confine your child's movements to carpet-less rooms while training, though if you have a particularly expensive (non-fitted) carpet or rug, then do anticipate the worst and remove it temporarily if you can.

Keep a bucket and cloth handy — a very dilute detergent solution should be sufficient. You can use a little bleach if you're quite sure you're using a small enough amount not to take the colour out of your carpet or flooring, or affecting the surfacing in any way (see page 138 for further information on getting rid of stains).

Also keep a pile of pants (and tights or trousers or whatever else you need) to hand, and encourage your child to get a replacement pair herself, and to put the soiled or wet articles where you tell her to.

1. Dr Robert Wilkins *The Power of the Potty* (General Practitioner, September 19, 1986)

# 7.

# OUT AND ABOUT — VISITS AND HOLIDAYS DURING TRAINING

Unless your child has been trained very quickly at a stage of relative maturity of the bladder, you are going to have to deal with 'calls of nature' after you have gone out of your front door, and consequently away from what has been up to now your nearest potty and toilet. This may mean problems if your child can't maintain sufficient control. You'll be able to gauge your child's ability to a certain extent by the length of time he can bear between needing the potty and actually opening his bowels and bladder. After all, there's more of a problem if he can't ever manage more than a second or two before it all happens. Nevertheless, given the challenge of *not* having the potty magicked up for him can sometimes help a child develop greater control.

You'll also face the problem of the not yet fully reliable child on outings if she's going through a particularly accident-prone stage, either at the very beginning of training or later...or even much later.

You might be happy, especially at the beginning, to just put nappies on your child to go out. This is the easiest solution in many ways, particularly if you haven't yet made a complete transition to 'no nappies' in the house. There are alternatives to this at a later stage, and parents develop their own strategies. These may give you some ideas.

'It's a good idea to have a mental list of all toilets in town as well as friends' houses en route'

*John*

'I took a potty everywhere until the twins were almost

three as they could never tell me they wanted to go in time for me to find a loo'

*Sophie*

'At first, I used to put a disposable nappy pad in his pants when we went out in the car, really for my benefit rather than his, as he was very quickly out of nappies once he made his mind up'

*Roz*

'We had accidents when we went out, but I just took some pants wherever we went and accepted the need for them.'

*Pamela*

'We had one outing a week after starting potty-training involving a bus journey of about 30 minutes. I took a towelling nappy and a polythene bag — and when he needed a wee I just held the nappy in the appropriate place'

*Joan*

'I took the potty with us at first, and then the toilet seat. I always had a change of clothing and I kept a plastic bag on the buggy seat to protect it.'

*Jean*

'I made sure both my children got used to the toilet from the very start and this made outings a lot easier than they would otherwise have been.'

*Gill*

Protecting the buggy seat (as Jean did) is a good idea, as not all buggy seats are removable for washing. The same applies to car seats. (Naturally you'll be aware of the dangers of plastic bags and not leave your child alone with one in reach.)

Disposable nappy pads (Roz's suggestion) are less easy to buy now all-in-one stick-on disposables have almost taken over because they're generally more efficient at the task of giving full protection. However, if you *can* get the pads (they're known as 'insert nappies' in the trade) they are useful for blotting the occasional accident. They are certainly less bother to put on and off than a proper nappy, disposable or terry, as you can quickly put one down inside the pants your child is already wearing, just before you go out. An alternative, although rather more clumsy, is to cut a towelling nappy into four and use one of the quarters, folded into three to make an oblong-shape, as a pad.

I'm not sure how widely applicable is Joan's suggestion of the strategically-placed nappy when on public transport, but for the odd occasion only it seems like a possibility. Not all children would find it acceptable, however, and presumably you'd need to be in a fairly private seat unless you are feeling pretty brazen.

Having a change of clothing is essential if there's any chance of you not getting to a loo or potty in time. Just pants won't be enough for boys, or for girls in tights and/or trousers, as their outer clothes will probably be wet, too. The handiest solution is always to have a pair of pull-on pyjama trousers rolled up in the bottom of your bag, together with pants and socks (pyjama bottoms these days look sufficiently like jogging trousers to pass perfectly well as such in an emergency).

Your child is bound to ask to go to the loo, or to use the potty you've brought, at an inconvenient time — in a shop where you know there are no public facilities, on a bus, on the motorway, in the high street... the list is endless. At times, yes, he may be asking when the need isn't there, or when he knows it's awkward. Most times, you'll just have to accept the request as genuine and do your best to act as quickly as possible.

In a department store, make your way to the nearest public convenience and if there's a queue you know will mean a wait that's unacceptable to your child, then don't be embarrassed about pushing in. 'I'm sorry — can my daughter/son go next? He/she's really desperate!' said with an apologetic smile will usually have people making way for you sympathetically. In a supermarket or shop where there are no public loos, then ask an assistant if you can use the staff facilities. It's rare that they'd prefer a puddle on the floor rather than allow you access. On past occasions, I've found the glimpse this gives me behind the scenes is illuminating. I don't think dirty toilets, with no soap or hot water in the basin or towels are appropriate in a food shop, for example — nor do I think it's right that boxes and cartons of food items should actually be stored in the toilets but this does go on, unfortunately.

Anywhere people work — libraries, bus depots, banks, building societies and so on — will have staff loos, in fact, and you shouldn't mind asking to use them on behalf of your child. Restaurants and cafes are of course obliged to have public ones.

In the street itself is a different matter. You can dive into the nearest place — shop, cafe, whatever — and ask. Or you may have to find a drain down an alleyway or side street and have your child urinate al fresco. This is only acceptable for passing water, of course, and you'll just have to hope your child won't want to pass an emergency bowel motion. Fortunately, he will be able to hang on better by this stage when he wants to open his bowels, and probably long enough for you to conjure up facilities from somewhere. If not, he won't be the first child to stagger home with messy pants, or to find a toilet too late and have to be cleaned up. These things you have to accept as a parent, too!

## Holidays

Holidays involve two possible problem areas for the newly-trained and semi-trained child: the travelling, and the unfamiliar place to stay.

During your journey, both going and returning, it's likely that you'll have to stop (if you go by car) more frequently than you are used to, for your child's sake. Obviously you'll try and make sure she visits the lavatory before you set off and at every scheduled stop thereafter, but these may not be enough. Use what you have already learnt about the sort of drinks that stimulate your child's bladder, and cut down on them or restrict them by not actually offering them while travelling. The lidded potty (see page 44) is useful, especially if your child needs to pass a bowel motion somewhere where you can't conveniently empty and rinse the potty afterwards. (Remember to have toilet paper and baby-wipes handy in the car — not at the bottom of someone's suitcase.)

Travelling by aeroplane you'll have toilets nearby, in the airport and on the plane itself. Queues can arise, though, especially on short-haul flights, so embark on the polite queue-barging routine on page 55. On a train, second-class carriage toilets are small and non-too clean. A fussy child may need to use the bigger, usually cleaner, first-class toilets (no, I don't mean you to buy a first-class ticket, just to use the loos in that part of the train. I don't *think* they can prosecute you for paying second, and 'going' first).

While you're away from home, some children might regress slightly (or even a lot) just because they're slightly disorientated and need to get used to the place you keep the potty, and where the loo is (or it may not affect your child at all, of course, one way or the other). Unfamiliar toilets can make a child very unhappy and lead to a downright refusal to use them.

'We were camping one year and had to use the toilet-block on the site. Richard had just progressed from using the potty to using the loo all the time, and we'd left the potty at home — but for five whole days he refused to use those loos for a poo. Naturally, he became very constipated. The loos were very mucky, it's true. The next few years we always paid special attention to the cleanliness and the design of the toilets before we decided to stay anywhere.'

*Rachel*

Situations like these — for example, where your child doesn't like the sound of the flush, or where the loo is outside in the yard or it's just 'different' in some unspecified way — will need a lot of extra reassurance from you, and an acceptance of his worry rather than a mockery of it. You could go back to the potty, or always promise to hold your child's hand while he uses the lavatory, or keep the door open (or shut).

# 8.

# WHEN ALL ELSE FAILED — STORIES OF UNEXPECTED SUCCESS

Sometimes parents feel they are making very little headway with training, and are tempted to put their child back into nappies as a recognition that the time is not yet right. However, something they then do, or something that happens coincidentally, becomes a breakthrough, confirming that the child was on the verge of control after all. Here's some examples that may give you ideas for your own child.

'I was rather tired of wet pants and quite ready to give up, then I saw some knickers with the My Little Pony characters on them in our local market. Sara was, and is, crazy on My Little Pony and I bought her a couple of pairs. She needed very little convincing that it would be a shame to get My Little Pony wet and from that time on she's hardly ever wet herself.'

*Julie*

'Katie's nappy fell off in the street one day. When we got home she demanded to wear pants from then on.'

*John*

'I discovered Lizzie's until then hidden passion for Ribena. Once I told her she could have some for every performance in the potty she really turned the corner to success. During this time we went in a supermarket, and she pointed gleefully to the Ribena on the shelf. "Potty juice! Potty juice!" she said delightedly!'

*Harriet*

'My health visitor suggested I put a nappy over the potty before my son used it. To my surprise it worked, and he happily sat on it and wee'd. Over the next week I gradually moved the nappy to the back of the potty and then removed it completely. I've had no wet or dirty nappies, day or night since. I never believed it could be so easy.'

*Heather*

'I'd had a couple of attempts at training my daughter but had met with screaming and an absolute refusal to sit on the potty, though I was certain she knew what was expected of her. I put the potty away in the end and decided not to do anything further for a few more months. Then one evening when she was 21 months old we went out to visit friends. They had a four-year-old daughter who disappeared on several occasions to go to the toilet closely followed by my daughter. She was obviously fascinated. When we got home she came to me holding herself underneath and showing an obvious desire to "go". She's now just over two, and from that day to this she's been clean and dry day and night and always uses the toilet.'

*Glenys*

'I'd had a right performance trying to train Thomas so I didn't feel like bothering trying to pot his younger sister Carly until she was two. When I did try, she was quite good, but then she began wetting. I put her straight back into nappies. Then, finally, Thomas became clean and dry at the age of $3\frac{1}{2}$, and Carly wanted to be like him. She asked for the pot again and was completely clean and dry within a fortnight.'

*Edith*

'Bobby idolized his big seven-year-old brother Peter. I'd had no success in getting Bobby out of nappies until Peter one day looked at him scornfully and said "stinky boy!" That was it — no more nappies.'

*Irene*

# 9.

# 'OVER-NIGHT SUCCESS' — HOW TO GET RID OF NIGHT-TIME NAPPIES

I'm dealing with night-time control separately, mainly because it seems, on the whole, to be achieved separately from day-time control. However, this isn't always the case. Some children (like Caroline on page 29) are dry and clean at night at the same time as they are dry and clean during the day, without anything special being done to achieve this. It can happen that night-time control actually comes before day-time control (see Mary's story on page 30) though this is unusual. The majority of parents in my survey reported that their children remained in nappies at night after they'd stopped wearing them in the day-time. This was obviously because they didn't feel control was adequate — a full bladder wouldn't be guaranteed to wake a child from sleep, at least not in time to stop a wet bed. (Some children who are trained in the day still have a day-time nap of an hour or two, and need a nappy on then too, at least at first.)

The approaches to night-time wetting during this stage differ. Active intervention in some form happens more often than a 'wait and see' policy, although many parents do take a back seat, and stop thinking about it all. This must be at least partly because a child who's trained in the day is socially acceptable, but there's not the same pressure from outside observers regarding night-training. Nevertheless, nappies worn beyond the age of four or five, even at night, are probably babyfying, seen through the eyes of the four or five-year-old. Manufacturers are producing some very large 'child size' disposable nappies, and the supermarkets are stocking them, which is a great help for those children still wearing nappies, and larger toddlers, whom terry nappies hardly fit.

The following quotations reflect what most parents do, or don't do.

'Amy stayed in night nappies for a short while, and just became dryer as time went on, and I left them off.'
*Gill*

'I lifted my son and took him to the toilet every night at about 11 pm, and I never let him have a drink after 6 o'clock.'
*Jean*

'When Laurie had been clean and dry in the day for about four months she asked if she could stop wearing a nappy at night. I complied, and she was dry more or less straight away.'
*Lena*

'Both my sons woke up frequently during the night until they were four or five, and each time they woke I encouraged them to go to the loo.'
*Barbara*

'When Paul insisted on doing without a nappy at night, at two years five months, we let him, but there were lots of wet beds. We quickly phased out his bedtime juice and gave him the choice — either a dry bed or a nappy, we didn't mind which. He chose the dry bed, and it took about a month for him to become 100 per cent reliable. Lifting is a waste of time — he learnt control because he wanted to. I reckon he'd sussed out that nappies are for babies and he wanted to be different from his baby sister.'
*Maggie*

'At $2\frac{1}{2}$, he's "drying out" slowly. His nappy is dry about every other morning, and I think I'll let him progress at his own rate without doing anything.'
*Alison*

'We would have had wet beds every time with Sam if we

hadn't restricted his drinks at bedtime, and lifted him each night, which we did for three years or so. However, he's now 7½ and we still tend to make sure he doesn't drink a lot before going to bed.'
*Dorothy*

'William's been dry in the day for a few months, but I still put a disposable on at night. I don't care how long he needs one — I'd rather change a nappy than a bed.'
*Gwen*

'We didn't consider Jon's night nappies to be a problem, but we were relieved when he finally did become dry. Staying with friends whose four-year-old didn't wear a nappy acted as a spur to him and to us. When we came home we started a star chart[1] which had him dry at night within two weeks.'
*Maxine*

'After she'd produced dry nappies for a little while, I left them off, and just lifted her when we went to bed for the next few months.'
*Wendy*

'We lifted both the children at night until they were about 3½. Then I put the potty by the bed and they used it by themselves.'
*Margaret*

'Lifting' is widely practised. It involves getting the child out of bed and getting him to pass water and then putting him back to bed again. It's often stated that waking the child up is an essential element in this process, though parents commonly lift their somnolent son or daughter and practically sleepwalk him or her to the lavatory where he or she urinates more or less still asleep, and they then put the child back to bed. The idea behind waking the child is so that the child emphatically *doesn't* pee in his sleep. After all, this is exactly what you want him to unlearn. You want him to wake up with the sensation of a full bladder, and to wake up sufficiently to get himself out of bed, hanging on to the urine the while, and across the landing or wherever to the toilet. Alternatively, you want him to sleep through the night undisturbed by his bladder. Lifting while he's asleep gets you nowhere nearer that situation.

On the other hand, there are children who are deep sleepers, and it is very difficult to wake them up without actually upsetting them. If you really reckon that lifting is saving wet beds, and you can't wake your child up without actually causing him distress or giving you both a subsequently broken night, then the practicalities of the situation may be that you'll continue lifting without waking. In the long-term, however, you'll have to consider whether your strategy isn't postponing the day when night-time wetting actually ceases.

A potty in the room is helpful to some children, though it can make the room smell, as you probably can't ask your child to empty and rinse it in the bathroom immediately after use (if he can do this he might as well go to the toilet anyway instead). Urine hanging about for hours, undealt with, seems to 'hang' in the air — and you also run the risk of the full potty being kicked over the following morning as your child gets out of bed.

What about restricting fluids? This can be a further way of helping your child's chances of a dry bed in the morning. It doesn't actually help with control, as when that is achieved it wouldn't actually matter how much was drunk — she'd wake to urinate anyway. But it's clear that a wet bed is uncomfortable and unpleasant for everyone, and giving the body less fluids to process means less work for the kidneys and bladder — and less chance of an accident. Do be careful your child isn't actually made to go to bed thirsty, however. You may have to make sure she has a good drink at teatime so she won't want such a large one later on.

It's sensible to expect the occasional accident, no matter whether you attempt to hurry night-time dryness or not. A waterproof mattress-cover, or sheet, under the bottom sheet is a practical measure — wiping urine from a mattress isn't easy, as it just soaks straight through, and it doesn't take many soakings to make the mattress smell and actually rot it.

Some children seem happy enough wetting their night nappies if you don't make any objections, and though one approach is to wait until you have a series of dry nappies before leaving them off altogether, your child may need a direct exhortation from you instead.

'I'd left day-time training until comparatively late. Rory took the initative himself, with my encouragement, at about $2\frac{1}{4}$. His nappies were still soaking every morning a year later, and I just did what I'd done with my first at this stage — I told him he was getting to be a big boy, and that soon he'd be able to go without a nappy. A couple of days later I didn't put a nappy on him and he's been dry almost every night since then.'
*Yvonne*

It can seem as though continuing to put nappies on your child is giving him permission to empty his bladder into them. If the ability to exercise control is there, it needs to be activated by taking away the safety net at times!

On average, night-time dryness happens at about the age of three, though there are plenty of perfectly normal children who are dry later than that with no long-term delay or problems. You can see more detailed figures in Chapter 11. Early-trained children, with regard to day-time control, tend to be dryer at night sooner than later-trained children. There are intensive methods for night training, however, (see page 108).

Opening the bowels unconsciously, that is while actually asleep, is extremely unusual beyond toddler hood. It's not uncommon, though, for a child to wait until he's got a night nappy on before passing a motion, or even do it in the morning before you've had a chance to take the nappy off. You can read about coping with this on page 123.

1. For more details about star charts and their application see page 101.

# 10.

# SPECIAL SITUATIONS — TWINS, THE HANDICAPPED CHILD.

**Twins**

Twins don't have to be 'harder' to train than singletons. The process is exactly the same, though the mothers I heard from tended to leave any formal training rather later than most mothers. This is because caring for twin toddlers is quite hard work in itself — exhausting, even — and the chance of anything that complicates matters isn't exactly seized.

Parents of twins will find this book as relevant as anyone else, but a few words of extra encouragement may help if you aren't looking forward to twice the number of wet pants and trousers and floors as everyone else.

When asked to look back on the toddlerhood of their twins, parents admit to being 'over anxious.'[1] This is because they find it difficult to cope with the excess of laundering and tend 'to hurry toilet training. This only delayed the process and caused too many frustrating moments'[2]. Once one twin makes progress, though, parents of twins notice that he or she may lead the other on which is useful. It's almost essential for your twins to have a potty each of course. You can take advantage of the close daily proximity of your twins and hope that they want to copy each other.

'We had one disastrous attempt at potty-training when they were 20 months. I put the pot away the minute it looked like making more work rather than less and it didn't emerge until they were over two. Andrea quickly got the hang of it, and I started giving her a Smartie every time she used the pot. Mark couldn't bear the idea of her getting a Smartie and not him... and after two days deprivation he rushed to use the potty and used it properly.'

*Kathleen*

'I've had four children, including the twins, and I didn't start to potty-train any of them until they were two. This worked well with the twins — Rosie was quicker than Jack and she was dry at night first too.'

*Celia*

A particularly practical and well-written book on twins,[3] which (like this one) uses the experiences of real-live parents and children, points out that twins are indeed aware of each others' capabilities and control while potty-training — but in some cases there may be a deal of difference between the ages at which progress is made. 'If one twin is ahead... it is very important to play down expressions of pleasure, particularly when the other twin is within earshot, even if he does appear to be totally unconcerned.... Each time the achieving child is praised, the other may take it as a reproach, which may in turn create unnecessary tension and set him back considerably'.[4] The pleasure you express needs to be low key, say the authors. They add that night-time nappies may be resented by the twin who's still in them. If the other twin is dry at night sooner, the nappy-wearing twin may insist on pyjamas only. This is a matter of your own judgement — wet beds (hopefully temporary) or a bit of a battle putting the nappy on the reluctant twin. If you do keep the twin in a nappy, it's sensible to explain to him that it won't be long before he'll be able to do without, as well.

Parents of triplets and quads (or more) will probably want to delay toilet-training as well, though if you're using terry-towelling nappies the prospect of not having to wash 15 or 20 nappies every day must be an attractive one.

## The handicapped child

The child who is mentally or physically disabled in some way does represent a special situation for parents. These days stress is placed on the aim of allowing all children to fulfill their potential and to become as able as possible to live within the community, as happily as possible. The vast majority of handicapped children live with their families, and this is especially true of younger ones. Professional guidance and support is available to varying degrees, depending on the health and social service provision in your area, and many young handicapped children will be given special educational help if it's needed, either in a special school or within mainstream (i.e. ordinary) schools.

Toilet-training can be an especially important step for a handicapped child as it is so vital socially, it greatly increases his or her independence and it gives the opportunity for a measure of responsibility. If you are already in touch with helping or supportive agencies, either through the health service or through your child's school, then ask for information and advice on training too.

Mentally handicapped children may take significantly longer than children of normal intelligence to reach bowel and bladder control. However, if there is no additional physical disability, the aim can certainly be to teach the child to recognize and respond to the usual physical signs of need quite independently of an adult. Some parents find the process is just as quick as would be expected with any other child. One mother has written of her daughter who has Downs Syndrome:

'Jessie at two was nappy-free during the day, and by three at night as well'.[5]

Much of the advice given in this book will be applicable to mentally handicapped children, and it may be that you need to be especially patient, and to involve other people more consistently in the training process. This may be inevitable, anyway, if your child is at school when the training is going on.

Two American researchers (who wrote the book mentioned on page 29) have developed a very intensive programme for toilet-training the handicapped. In fact, their ideas started there, and were later adopted for use by other children and their parents.[6] The programme is also used in a modified form for bed-wetting[7] and this too has been put forward as applicable to all children with night-time wetting problems (see page 108). Their results are impressive, and although the programme demands a particularly high level of committment from the adults involved — parents and teacher — the evidence is that this method can work where others have failed. A real-life example of success with this method is described in a parents' handbook, written by a psychologist specializing in mental handicap[8]. It follows a morning with a nine-year-old boy who had never been clean and dry for no really obvious reason. The programme used was very intensive, concentrating 'full time on toiletting, and including many frequent regular checks on pants, extra liquids for the child to drink, frequent trips to the toilet, massive re-inforcement for success and some mild punishment for accidents.'[8] In this particular case the reward for appropriate behaviour was a bar of chocolate, awarded for dry pants and the successful use of the toilet, and mild punishment was getting the child to wash out his own wet pants in cold water.

Physically handicapped children may have problems which inhibit them getting to the toilet or the potty in time, day or night. Even children with just a minor degree of neurological impairment, showing up as 'clumsiness', may find it difficult to gain control because the physical actions involved in sitting on the loo and coping with clothing are so awkward to co-ordinate. Children who are hearing-impaired, if not actually deaf, are likely to have language delay, which will slow up their ability to understand, cooperate and communicate with you about using the potty. Blind and sight-impaired children have obvious difficulties too with using the potty or the toilet correctly and will need special teaching to overcome these.

Many handicapped children are disabled in more than one way, of course, and careful assessment of their abilities and limitations as individuals will help you and the professionals involved to judge the right time and way to teach about bowel and bladder control. The major charities concerned with handicap often have useful information focusing on this very topic, and can in any case put you in touch with other parents whose experience will be valuable to you. I'd especially recommend the Disabled Living Foundation, who have a great deal of information about making toileting easier for adults and children with a handicap, plus up-to-date facts about aids for incontinent people and for older and/or handicapped children who are not yet toilet trained.[9]

1. Judi Linney *Multiple Births – preparation, birth, managing afterwards* (John Wiley & Sons, 1983)
2. ibid.
3. Elizabeth Friedrich and Cherry Rowland *The Twins Handbook* (Robson Books 1983)
4. ibid.
5. Elsa Parris *Jessie — the story of a very special child* (Good Housekeeping magazine, December 1986)
6. N.H. Azrin, R.M. Foxx (1973) *Dry pants — a rapid method of toilet training children* (Behaviour Research and Therapy 11, 435–442)
7. N.H. Azrin, T.J. Sneed, R.M. Foxx (1973) *Dry bed: a rapid method of eliminating bedwetting (enuresis) of the retarded* (Behaviour Research and Therapy 11, 427–434)
8. Janet Carr *Helping your Handicapped Child* (Penguin 1980)
9. Disabled Living Foundation, 380–384 Harrow Road, London W9 2HU. Telephone 01–289 6111

# PART TWO: PROBLEMS

We've already dealt in Part One with some of the minor setbacks every parent should aim to take as inevitable during the training period, and you'll find some very specific queries answered in the Questions and Answers section at the end of the book. Here in Part Two, we'll deal with more long-standing hold-ups and difficulties, and tell you how far you can expect to deal with them yourself, and when to seek outside help, together with what to expect from it if you do.

# 11.

# DELAYS IN ACHIEVING BLADDER AND BOWEL CONTROL

Any problems with bowel and bladder control may be physical or emotional in origin. In many cases, as we'll see, the problem may be caused by a physical difficulty and then be complicated by emotional factors. The reverse is also true — the problem starts off by being an emotional (or psychological) one, and then a true physical element may develop and remain after the emotional difficulty has been dealt with. Knowing, or being able to guess at, the cause of a problem can be only a part of the story, however, and may offer no more than an insight, rather than a practical solution. Knowing when *not* to do anything, and when to stop worrying and just start waiting for time alone to solve the problem isn't always easy for parents, who so often feel guilty about their children's difficulties or delays. It's as if you feel you *should* be able to do something to help the situation, and when you don't seem to be able to, it can be very distressing — and you feel under real pressure from all sides.

Let's take by far the commonest problem first — simple delay in achieving bowel and/or bladder control. 'Delay' is a pretty subjective assessment of course, and will depend on your own expectations, or, (sometimes, unfortunately, even more important) the expectations of other people. Many parents get very upset when their child doesn't seem to cotton on.

'Our daughter is now two years five months and still not trained. I find it heartbreaking when we go to toddler group and there's 18 month olds asking mummy to take them to the loo and we're still struggling.'

*Diane*

'When Martin was two and still not out of nappies, I was beginning to get desperate — especially when all my friends' children were already trained.'

*Marie*

'For two years, no matter how often I potted him he would have innumerable accidents in between, and in the end I found I was getting really angry with him which I knew was wrong.'

*Cath*

'At two years eight months, Ben refuses to stop wearing nappies... I am beginning to despair.'

*Marcia*

At this early stage, it's not the child who has the problem, it's the parents. 'Heartbreaking' when a toddler isn't as quick to get the message as others? 'Despair' at a refusal to give up nappies? Come off it! There are a lot of really tragic situations that can befall a family, and a slow-to-be-trained child isn't one of them. If you feel this way, ask yourself if you are over-reacting and giving far too much importance to this single aspect of toddlerhood. I know as much as any other mother of small children how tiring, how infuriating, how (sometimes) *boring* their day-to-day care can be — but that's not the whole story. Parenting toddlers can be hugely enjoyable and rewarding as well. But once you start focusing on an area that's especially tiring, infuriating and boring (as unsuccessful, long-lasting training can be), then you risk eclipsing all the good bits. Surely life, and childhood, is too short for that?

Most children under about three aren't at all bothered about being clean and dry or being seen in nappies. Once they see that you are, however, it's easy for them to turn this whole area into a battle ground. It may be a noisy or aggressive battleground — some toddlers scream when they see the potty; some mothers end up smacking far more often than they really think they ought to. It may be a more quiet, subtle battle of wills which you the parent can't actually win. After all, you *can't* force your child to urinate, or to move his bowels when you say he has to. You can try, and dire threats may have a short-term effect in some cases. But ultimately, they are *his* bowels, and *his* bladder, and he may eventually use whatever control he develops in his way alone.

In Chapter 6 *Coping with Accidents* on page 48, there are some practical ideas which may help to ease the situation. However, a change of attitude on your part may be far more important, if you feel things have become problematical. Take the pressure off yourself for a start, by accepting the wetting/soiling situation as *normal*. If you find that difficult to accept, take a look at the statistics quoted below. And if it's still hard to swallow, then at least try to pretend you're not greatly bothered, for your child's sake.

Much is said about children being able to pick up tension and worry, even if adults try to hide it. I think this is perhaps over-stated. Children can't read your mind (not until they're at least six or seven anyway!) and a determined act of unconcern as described on page 51 will be quite convincing as long as it's *consistently* maintained. It's possible that you'll convince yourself in the process that this is actually what you feel.

The point is that if you get to a stage when training is coming between you and your child, if progress is slow enough to irritate you, or even to rouse you to anger, or to make you guilty, or otherwise unhappy, then stop what you're doing, and re-think your approach. You might decide to put the whole idea of training on to the back-burner for a while, and return to full-time nappies. Or you can look through the suggestions in Chapters 2 and 8 and begin all over again on a new footing.

One thing contributing to your anxiety about training may be an underlying lack of confidence in yourself and an erroneous feeling of inferiority to other mothers. It's really hopeless to compare your child's progress with that of other people's sons and daughters. Just as most people surely accept that different children have different rates of progress in walking and talking without a 'slow' or 'quick' rate reflecting well or badly on the parents, control of bowel and bladder in the early years shows a wide variability, too. It's not a race... it's not a mark of good mothering... or innate intelligence... or 'niceness'.

Negative feelings about the process won't help you cope — and one highly negative feeling is suspecting that other people are wondering why you haven't yet trained your child. Some mothers report that they've received actual adverse comments about the situation from others. Kaye, for example, whose son was in nappies at three, wrote: 'I came in for a lot of criticism from other people who felt he should have been out of nappies earlier'.

Not everyone can summon up the confidence to go against other people's opinions, or to counter direct criticism with the calm assertion that you're doing what you believe is right for you and your family — or the less calm assertion that other people can darn well mind their own business! Personally, I think anyone who feels they have the right to tell you when your child should be trained has a right cheek. Well-meaning concern from family and friends is different but it still needs the same self-confident reactions from you.

Don't let the guilt that every parent can feel about a whole range of issues make you attempt to demonstrate what a perfect, organized, in-control Supermum you are. Don't allow yourself to feel that a three-year-old in nappies is letting you down. Instead, ask yourself what is more important: a relaxed, happy relationship with your child, or a daily struggle to maintain an attempt to impose your wishes on him?

A belief that your child will be trained eventually is vital, of course. One mother told me her doctor had said her two-year-old 'would *never* be trained' if she didn't get him out of nappies soon; another said her mother kept making predictions about the three-year-old needing to go to school in nappies. What nonsense!

Even if you and your child are happy about his/her rate of progress, there are playgroups and nursery units which have a sort of condition of entry insisting that all children starting there must be trained.

'I've not bothered too much about the fact that Becky still needs reminding about the toilet — if she's not reminded she just wets and soils herself. But she's been offered a place at nursery school and if I can't get her properly trained the place will be withdrawn.'

*Shelagh*

This is actually rather unfair. I do sympathize with teachers and playgroup leaders who feel their attentions and skills are not best used in toileting or potting, but so many children of pre-school age have accidents that to use this as a means to exclude children who would otherwise benefit is rather arbitrary. Naturally, staff would prefer all children to be trained — that's understandable — but if the nursery or playgroup make it a rigid pre-condition, I'd wonder how many more of their policies fail to acknowledge different rates of development and different needs. There could be a case for looking around for more flexible pre-school provision. Alternatively, a word with the staff may persuade them to take on your 'problem child' in the hope that seeing a group of other children who are trained will make the the crucial difference.

A possible way of making progress if you feel the 'training relationship' between you and your child is at breaking point, and you feel even a 'cooling off' period in nappies won't be enough to erase memories, is to pass the task onto someone else. Dad, or grandma, or even a considerably older brother or sister, may do in a weekend or a week's holiday what you've been gnashing your teeth over for months! The point is *not* that you're a wash-out as a mum, but that these other people are not emotionally involved with the idea of 'failure', nor have they had the demoralizing experience of getting nowhere fast (or slow) in the previous weeks or months.

### Some facts and figures
As for those statistics, a 1982 report looked at the day and night wetting of 706 three-year-olds in an outer London borough[1]. The author defined 'wet' during the day as being wet at least once a week. 'Dry' meant wetting less than once a week. It's important to acknowledge that 'wet' will also include children who wet very frequently, though this

result wasn't published in the report. 23 per cent of boys and 13 per cent of girls were wet by day. 55 per cent of boys and 40 per cent of girls were wet by night. With regard to soiling ('soilers' were defined as children who had soiled at least once during the previous month), 21 per cent of boys were 'soilers' and 11 per cent of girls. To quote the author, 'wetting at this age seems to be largely under the control of maturational factors' — in other words, it depends on whether the child has grown out of wetting or not.

No really significant links were found between wetting at three and other factors such as social class, housing conditions, family stresses, relationships with brothers and sisters. The study didn't aim to look very closely at soiling but the very high incidence of its occasional happening certainly indicates that it's still fair to call it 'normal' in children of three.

It's interesting to note the consistently higher proportion of boys still wetting or soiling at this age, too. There's no real physical or anatomical reason for the adage that boys are harder and slower to train than girls. It's more likely to be at least partly caused by two phenomena: firstly, the comparative slowness of the rate that boys mature (in all sorts of ways) relative to girls. Remember, girls reach puberty on average a year or two ahead of boys. Secondly, the way girls tend to be more 'biddable' than boys throughout childhood and adolescence is likely to mean they are more willing to co-operate with training.

You could spend a life time speculating — and many people have done just that — whether this character trait is there because females are born with it or whether it's induced because of the way baby girls are brought up and the expectations parents have of them. The fact that this trait is there, however, is underlined in the same survey, which finds that there is an association between day wetting in boys and more generalized behaviour problems. 18 per cent of boys *without* a behaviour problem were wet during the day; 43 per cent of those *with* a behaviour problem were wet. There was no link between behaviour problems and wetting in girls, fewer of whom had behaviour problems anyway. I think it's reasonable to conclude from this that boys tend to be more 'difficult' than girls at the pre-school stage at least, and that their wetting is actually likely to be part of a series of generally immature behaviour patterns and responses. Take heart, mothers of sons — in so many cases, your boys are just slower to grow up than their sisters!

1. Kirk Weir (1982) *Night and Day Wetting among a population of three-year-olds* (Developmental Medicine and Child Neurology, 24, 479–484)

# 12.

# PHYSICAL PROBLEMS

Any general practitioner has queues of people at every surgery who have some malfunctioning of the bowels or the 'waterworks', and common difficulties like constipation and diarrhoea are particularly prevalent in young children. On the whole, there's usually nothing desperately serious wrong, though you do need to seek medical advice if you're at all worried about your child, (this book's not a medical manual, and I'm not a doctor). However, there are certain bits of factual information which are useful to know; home treatment, administered with common sense, can save you and your doctor, not to mention your child, time and hassle. Nevertheless, you'll need to supplement the information here with advice from your health visitor or your doctor. They know you and your child and will be able to make a more accurate diagnosis, having asked you questions to complete the picture. The chances are you'll find reassurance with or without actual treatment, and possibly some advice on preventing a re-occurence of the problem.

With babies, my advice would be to go to the doctor sooner rather than later as babies can become ill more quickly than toddlers or older children.

### Constipation
Constipation is defined as the production of dry, hard, difficult-to-pass stools. It usually means the stools are passed infrequently — though passing infrequent stools in itself does not necessarily mean constipation, as it's the type and texture that are important. In breastfed babies — fully breastfed babies, that is — constipation is virtually

unknown. Though the baby may go several days between stools, the motion produced (eventually) is very soft. Bottle-fed babies may get constipated, possibly as a result of incorrectly mixed feeds, or dehydration. Always seek your health visitor's advice (you can usually telephone her) or see your doctor. You may be advised to increase your baby's fluid intake or to give some fruit juice. Once mixed feeding starts — that is, when foods other than milk are introduced — it's not uncommon for babies to get a bit 'bunged up' as their digestive systems may find certain new foods hard to cope with, and their fluid intake may decrease, too. Again, if the problem persists, get advice and make a mental note of the foods you think may have contributed to the problem.

In a toddler or child, constipation is primarily caused by a diet that's too low in fluids and/or dietary fibre.

Unless you've just arrived from Mars, or not read any newspapers or magazines or watched TV for the last 10 years, you don't need me to tell you which foods contain fibre — but I'll remind you just the same. Fibre is the nutritional buzz word of the 1980s, and the lack of it is thought to be responsible for a quite staggering selection of physical disorders. Few experts doubt that it's needed to maintain a healthy bowel, though its other possible benefits have yet to be accepted as fully proven.

Basically, fibre is formed from the cell walls of plants (fruit, vegetables, grains) and it's needed to bulk out the stool, to make the water content of the stool sufficiently high for comfort. The standard Western diet of highly-refined processed foods has less fibre than even a generation ago, and you may have to make a special effort to make sure you and your family choose food items that have enough. The foods you'll be looking for are fruit and vegetables (cooked, if at all, with much of their skins intact, and not reduced to a mush in gallons of boiling water) and whole grains. This will mean choosing wholemeal bread, and opting for brown pasta and rice at least occasionally, and looking at other less widely available grains too (for more ideas see page 127). There are plenty of whole-grain breakfast cereals around, many of them aimed specifically at children. Some children seem to need more fibre in their diet than others to prevent constipation.

There's not a lot to be said in favour of giving children bran as a dietary supplement. This is to be avoided with toddlers, who will find it especially hard to digest. Children of all ages are likely to find its taste unpalatable, and it can cause a lot of wind and colicky-type pains. It's better to improve the over-all quality of your child's diet, and offer extra fruit and especially extra fluids, as lack of liquid intake can predispose to constipation. Normally, we drink when we're thirsty, and that, together with drinks we might have just because we like them, is sufficient. Again, though, some children need more fluid than others and you may need to supply your child with a drink when he hasn't actually asked for one, or make a drink an integral part of his meals, to keep him 'going'.

It's worth checking that a child prone to constipation isn't intolerant to certain foods. This would show up as a hard-to-pass stool on the day after the food has been eaten. For you to be confident that a particular food was to blame, you'd have to see the same reaction every time, and find that the constipation never happened when the suspected food was excluded from the diet. If you come to some sort of conclusion, you may find that it's merely a phase in your child's development, and that the same food re-introduced at a later date produces no problems at all. So a 'constipated reaction' to eggs, for example, wouldn't necessarily be life-long.

There could be a psychological aspect to your child's constipation, that could be described as 'fear of opening the bowels'. The child, consciously or unconsciously hangs on to the bowel motion because he doesn't want to let it go. He may fear it will hurt — if he's already constipated then this could be true. Hard, dry stools do hurt. He may have an anal fissure (see below) which will give him pain every time he opens his bowels. This hanging on in itself creates or aggravates the constipation, and of course leads to a worsening of the problem as the child is given more reason to hold back. The whole situation can become miserable for both parent and child.

'People who haven't experienced the problems wouldn't believe the way Joseph's constipation took over our lives. He only opened his bowels once every five days or so. He would start wanting to go on say, a Tuesday, and be 'niggly' and fractious; throughout Wednesday and Thursday he would get worse, and by the Friday he'd be unable to stay still for more than a few seconds and be in obvious pain. Eventually he would 'let go' and things would get better — and he'd be something like a normal happy three-year-old, until the cycle started again.'

*Penny*

Circumstances like these may need some form of intervention. Rather than forcing your child to sit on the potty or toilet and to damned well stay there until something happens — or else, it's probably kinder and more effective to break the cycle of 'constipation ... fear ... constipation' with treatment (and with possible dietary changes as outlined above) in order to allow a normal bowel action the chance to get established.

Hanging on until constipation results can be a clear result of a change in a child's routine or toilet habit, rather than fear of pain or discomfort.

'At two years 10 months, Hugh had been clean and dry for over a year. We were having some work done on the house and the workmen had to lay new plumbing. This meant there was a hole in the wall where the toilet was. Hugh refused to sit on the toilet for a poo, although wee'ing was okay — he could stand up for that. But he hung on and on — he wouldn't use the potty, or the toilet in anyone else's house either. Eventually we suggested a nappy, which he was happy to accept, and he got us to take it off to pass water. However, he still didn't open his bowels, and after seven or eight days he started having diarrhoea by-pass[1]. The doctor prescribed a laxative, and after 10 or 12 days he eventually 'succumbed', but the problem continued even when the hole in the wall was repaired.'

*Annie*

A similar tale of "loo resistance" is recounted on page 57.

Usually, once the cycle is broken, whether the hanging on is physical or emotional in its causes, life can get back on an even keel. But that's not always the case. Hugh in the previous report needed a daily dose of laxative for six months and even two years later, Annie had to keep an unobtrusive note of how often he went to the loo, and remind him to go if he allowed more than a couple of days between visits.

## Should laxatives be used?

Many people are rightly reluctant these days to take unnecessary medication and that goes for our children too. We know that a reliance on laxatives in particular can lead to the bowel becoming unable to work normally. However, as a short-term solution to the problem of constipation in children they are very valuable. Children with a long-standing underlying disorder that's become complicated with emotional factors may actually need laxatives for some time (for more discussion on this, see pages 115 and 138).

While therapy is underway, it may be important, as with Hugh, to keep the stool soft and easy to pass (which is the main function of most of the milder laxatives prescribed these days) to prevent problems building up again. These so-called 'stool softeners' are helpful and, on the whole, harmless.

Discuss your anxieties with your doctor, and don't give over-the-counter laxatives yourself without asking his advice. Occasionally, the doctor may decide to give an enema or a suppository. These are administered directly into the rectum — the enema is liquid, the suppository is a solid sort of tablet — and though apparently in other countries they're used as commonly as cough lozenges, in Britain we don't usually thrill to the idea. There may be a case for their use when the rectum is so grossly distended with faeces that have become virtually impossible to pass, but in the majority of cases oral laxatives will be sufficient.

## Anal fissure

This is a small split in the delicate mucous membrane of the anus. It is painful for a 'victim' to open the bowels as a result, and there may be some bleeding, too. The fissure is caused by a hard motion which tears the skin of the anus, and because the area is more or less moist all the time, healing can take a little while.

It's important that your child's motions remain soft and easy to pass if she has an anal fissure, otherwise the fissure is more likely to be opened again and the healing process will be delayed. Pay attention to her diet (see page 82), and be aware that the pain of bowel opening may lead to constipation if your child hangs on because of reluctance to defecate.

Don't worry about the bleeding — it's no more serious than bleeding from any small cut would be.

You can ask your health visitor or doctor about creams to buy in the chemist, which will help promote healing as well as easing the motion out if the cream is applied just before it's passed (or use a small dab of Vaseline instead which will lubricate the anus).

'Belinda hadn't ever been constipated to my knowledge, but at 6½ she started telling me it hurt when she opened her bowels. I got a fright when she told me there was blood on the loo paper, but of course I needn't have worried about that aspect of it. The fissure took weeks to heal properly. I've told her to let me know if she gets constipated again, and I always make sure I offer her a drink of juice with her breakfast. Left to herself she mightn't bother.'

*Ursula*

## Diarrhoea

At the other end of the spectrum as it were, is diarrhoea. This is the frequent passage of runny stools, often accompanied by pain and vomiting. Again, fully breastfed babies don't normally get it. Their stools are runny anyway, and may even have bits of mucus in them. As well as infrequent bowel motions being normal in a breastfed baby, it's also normal to have very frequent ones (my three children dirtied almost every nappy they wore for six months!) and even the occasional green stool in a contented thriving breastfed baby is no more than a sign of 'intestinal hurry'.

In a bottle-fed baby diarrhoea isn't uncommon, and it is probably caused by a bug (bottle-fed babies don't get the protection against illness that comes with breast milk, and feeding equipment can harbour bacteria). You should seek advice soon, and as soon as possible if the diarrhoea is accompanied by vomiting. (Vomiting in a breastfed baby needs investigating as well, though it's more likely to be overflow being regurgitated than anything more serious.) Small babies can become dehydrated very quickly, and if the baby is losing fluid at both ends so to speak, something needs to be done.

'D and V' as the doctors term diarrhoea and vomiting, can be hazardous to any young child if it's allowed to go on too long, and most sensible doctors will take your concern seriously. It can be one of the symptoms of a range of illnesses, as can diarrhoea on its own.

Small babies and toddlers may get diarrhoea as a reaction to a new food — just as when you note transient constipation as a reaction (see page 82), this is something you may remember and as a result avoid the offending foodstuff or restrict your child to small quantities of it for the time being.

Persistent diarrhoea can be a sign of intolerance to a certain food. (There may be other symptoms in a highly sensitive child, such as skin rashes, pains, difficult behaviour and even sleepiness.) Don't try to diagnose food intolerance yourself — you might suspect it, of course — without confirmation from a diet-minded doctor or a dietician. You will then be able to make the necessary adjustments to your child's diet without running the risk of allowing your child to go short of various important nutrients. In the case of a milk allergy, for instance, it could be harmful to remove all milk products from your child's diet without careful thought and advice to how the protein and the vitamins and minerals he'd normally be getting from milk could be substituted.

Some children get diarrhoea as a reaction to antibiotics they are taking.

Generally speaking, a child whose motions are diarrhoea –like (frequent and loose), but who is in otherwise good health and is developing well, is fine. This is certainly the case with what is sometimes called 'toddler diarrhoea'. This is actually quite common, and most family doctors are familiar with it.

'Timothy was really prolific in the bowels department! Up to the age of about three he would open his bowels anything up to four times a day. When he was between about one and two I used to have to take a clean pair of trousers for him wherever we went because he just used to explode and the nappy and plastic pants couldn't contain it. We had some *very* messy moments, I can tell you! He was, and is, perfectly healthy, and even now, at five, he has a couple of poos a day at least.'

*Ursula*

Toddler diarrhoea does ease off with time, though during the toilet-training period it can cause one or two problems as the bowel motions can arrive without as much warning as you might prefer.

**Urinary tract infections** are also common in young children. Symptoms include pain on passing water, frequency of passing water (difficult to be sure about this, of course, unless you notice a sudden change in the pattern of your child's needs for the potty or lavatory), constant dribbling of urine, cloudy or 'strong' urine, and urgency (when the need to pass urine is sudden and urgent). Sometimes there may be no obvious symptoms to do with the passing of urine, but your child may appear ill in other ways, too.

Urinary tract infections are usually caused by bacteria that normally live in the bowel — where they cause no harm — entering the urinary tract via the urethra. It's a lot easier for this to happen in girls than boys, partly because the urethra can so easily come into contact with the bowel motions because of the way the female genitalia are arranged, and partly because the urethra itself is much shorter in girls than in boys. One child care book states that infection of this sort is 10 times more common in girls than in boys[2]. Girls should always be taught to wipe their bottoms 'front to back' to reduce the risk of infection.

If you suspect a urinary tract infection in your child you should see your child's doctor. He may want to check for a physical abnormality (see below) and he may prescribe antibiotics to clear the infection. Children who wet during the day or during the night are sometimes found to have a urinary infection, but this is thought to be the result, rather than the cause, of the wetting. Once the infection is cleared, the wetting continues — a phenomenon recorded in several studies[3].

Boys sometimes develop an infection called balinitis underneath the foreskin. The symptoms are redness, and pain in passing urine. The treatment for this may not have to be antibiotics, but a simple attention to hygiene — the foreskin needs to be gently pulled back as far as it will go and washed and then dried at bath time.

**Physical abnormalities** may affect the way your child attains bowel or bladder control. Gross defects in the intestinal and urinary tracts are fortunately very rare, and these are usually spotted at birth. Less obvious problems may not be diagnosed until later. A tight foreskin in a boy may lead to repeated infections and the eventual need for circumcision. Hirschsprung's disease is a very rare congenital abnormality, but in its less severe forms it can show up as very bad constipation. It's a defect in the nerve supply to the bowel which leads to a failure of the intestine to contract as it normally would to pass the faeces downwards. The result is a 'bunging up' within the intestinal tract.

Hypospadias is a 'mis-placement' of the urethra in boys. The urethra normally opens at the tip of the penis; in hypospadias the opening is elsewhere on the underside of the penis. Producing a normally-directed stream of urine is not possible in any but the mildest cases, and surgery may be carried out to correct the defect, once the child reaches the age of about three.

1. See page 113
2. Drs Andrew and Penny Stanway *The Baby & Child Book* (Pan, 1983)

3. For example, I. Berg, D. Fielding, R. Meadow (1977) *Psychiatric disturbance, urgency and bacteriuria in children with day and night wetting* (Archives of Diseases in Childhood, 52, 651–657)

# 13.

# WETTING DURING THE DAY

Day-time wetting can be worrying. However, if the child has never been satisfactorily reliable about using the toilet, it can be a feature of normal delay in control even in four or five-year-olds, and the child seems to grow out of it.

Regular deluges when a whole bladder-full of urine is eliminated down the legs, are unusual, though. Beyond the age of three-and-a-half the majority of children will be aware of the strong sensation of a full bladder and will recognize the urge to pass water. The odd full-scale accident may still happen to any child when she feels nervous, frightened and puts off going to the lavatory because there isn't a decent one nearby or she's shy about asking to go.

'I remember when I was seven, the teacher asked me to recite a poem I was supposed to have learnt and hadn't. I was so terrified of her rage when I got up, I stood in paralysed silence as I soaked my legs and the floor, totally, uncontrollably. Even now, the memory of it makes me want to crawl away!'

*Viv*

Disasters of this sort are part of the scenery in every nursery and infants' class, even though they may only happen occasionally to individuals. All primary schools have a stock of spare knickers, socks and trousers.

It's when accidents like this happen again and again to a child that you need to ask yourself why, and perhaps seek professional advice.

The theory that day-wetters can't actually hold on to

# WETTING DURING THE DAY

much urine because their bladders are small could offer a partial explanation of the problem though it can't be all the story. Frequency — the need to urinate often — is seen in day-wetters, it's true, but this could also be explained by the fact that many day-wetters go to the loo more often because this is a way they or their parents, try to prevent the wetting.

It's been suggested that persistent day-wetters (who almost always wet at night too) have something wrong with the way their bladders respond, and the way their muscles are used. In other words the child isn't able to co-ordinate the need to urinate with the sphincter muscle and pelvic-floor muscles.[1] Using a technique called urodynamic biofeedback, researchers can measure the amount of pressure present in the bladder during urination, and exactly where and what is being exerted. For some reason, the technique of urinating 'properly' either hasn't been learnt by the child or it has been forgotten. The result is that the urine may not be fully eliminated, and it often happens that the bladder starts to contract at other times when the child isn't aware of feeling full. The urge is so strong at that point that these contractions can't be stopped, and the child has to dash to the loo, or else 'do it' there and then. It would seem that somehow or other the sequence of events of full bladder ... controlling of urge ... emptying of bladder has become impossible to rely on.

Some interesting work has been done teaching day-wetters to recognize when they are urinating incorrectly, with the use of this technique of urodynamic biofeedback. The muscle actions and bladder pressure during urination are 'read' by electrodes attached to the perineum and the results come up on a screen or a graph, giving a visual representation that the child can see. The doctors then teach the correct ways of relaxing and contracting the muscles and the child can see the difference on the screen or graph when she's doing it right. This gives her the opportunity to recognize, and put into practice every time, the proper actions.

The results of this particular study were good — out of 10 patients, eight were 'cured' and two showed an improvement. The problem with this technique is that it's time consuming. The child needs to stay in hospital where all the equipment is, and needs fairly intensive teaching over a period of a couple of days. It's unlikely that the techniques will be offered widely, though the knowledge that muscle control can be taught is helpful.

Some doctors use drugs to control urination, but most people would feel that long-term achievement of self-control is preferable. It's also been found that children who wet during the day as well as at night show more signs of psychiatric disturbance and problem behaviour than children who only wet at night,[2] though this *doesn't* mean that all children who wet during the day are disturbed. It may be a factor in some cases, and psychiatric or psychotherapeutic help may lead to a solution to the problem. There's the possibility, though, that day-time wetting is the *cause* of the disturbed behaviour, not the result, because of anxiety the child has developed about it.

However, children from families with severe relationship, financial, housing and social problems are more likely to wet during the day, without necessarily showing other strong evidence of disturbed behaviour. In one study of 129 families with multiple problems[3], as many as 6.3 per cent of the children were wet by day at the age of eight.

Day-wetting may not show up as a full regular flooding, but more like a frequent 'seepage' of urine, leading to permanently damp pants. This is very common in small children, and it is likely to be a symptom of immaturity as well as having an element of non-cooperation. The child can forget or ignore the sensation of a full bladder, or just not respond to it quickly enough, and the result is that some urine leaks out between visits to the lavatory, or it starts to leak before the child gets there. Being in soggy pants can lead to infections and a sore bottom as well as being inconvenient because of the extra washing. Sometimes you can encourage your child not to rush off the toilet once she thinks she's finished, but just to relax and wait a second or two to release the odd few drops of urine that may not have been eliminated. It could be helpful to try and improve voluntary control — not by urging a visit to the toilet every half-hour, but by reminding her to go at sensible times when she has the chance, like just before school, at break times during school and so on. Make sure any infection is regularly dealt with, as although (as we've seen on page 87) the infection may not have instigated the wetting, its presence will not help the 'cure'. Playing the whole thing down, and treating it as something you know will disappear eventually is far better than becoming angry or exasperated — or showing that that's how you feel.

1. E.C. Sugar, C.F. Firlit (1982) *Urodynamic biofeedback: a new therapeutic approach for childhood incontinence/infection* (Journal of Urology, 128, 1253—1258)
2. Berg et al op.cit. note 3, p.89.
3. A.F. Philp *Family Failure* (Faber and Faber, 1963)

# 14.

# BED-WETTING

The correct term for this is enuresis — and more specifically nocturnal enuresis, because it happens at night. It is common at *all* ages, right into and including adulthood — an estimated one per cent of adults wet the bed.

For some families it becomes a major problem. However, it's not always recognized as a phenomenon needing understanding, sympathy and help — practical help for the families concerned because of the extra work in washing and drying, and emotional help for the children themselves. There are some heartfelt accounts in my files from people who have had to deal with prolonged periods of bed-wetting. Some parents find the whole thing more difficult than others to cope with, and at its worst it starts to affect the whole way parents react to their child.

'I am a health lecturer, and I know from my professional experience that bed-wetting in my $3\frac{1}{2}$-year-old son is not in itself a problem. But the continued round of washing and drying sheets, duvets and pillows I find a real bind.'

*Trisha*

'I'm now 23, and up the age of 15 I wet the bed. I was sent to a specialist a number of times, but neither he nor my G.P. — who kept saying for years that I would 'grow out of it' — was any help. I always hated getting up for school because there would be the question, was the bed dry? Most of the time it wasn't, and we'd start the day with a row. When I met the boy who was to become my husband, it suddenly stopped. I haven't wet the bed since then. I have a daughter of my own now, and I hope she never goes through what I had to.'

*May*

'I wet the bed until I was 16. When I used to wake up soaking, it infuriated my father. He treated me like a puppy — rubbing my nose in my wet bed. I hated him for it. I was marched off to a clinic loads of times. They said I was lazy. My father got even more angry. I was given a buzzer alarm[1] but it didn't work. It woke me up and I'd go to the loo, but then the buzzer was switched off, and I'd wet again later. I now know I wasn't using it correctly. When I was 10, my father left home, and my mother just left me to it without allowing herself, or, me, to become too upset. In the holidays I used to stay with an aunt, who promised me a savings stamp for every dry night. She would also wake me up to go to the toilet at about midnight. This worked, and I never wet when I was there. It started again at home, though. Looking back, I think I wet the bed because of three reasons — the message that I needed to go to the toilet was never strong enough to wake me up; I was shy and insecure and felt neglected in a family of seven children; occasionally I'd dream I was on the toilet and I'd pass water then. It stopped shortly after I moved in with my boyfriend. For a month we'd wake to a wet bed at about 2 am. We'd change the sheets and go back to sleep, and then it just stopped. I suppose deep down I felt safe.'

*Terry*

'I stopped wetting the bed regularly at 17, but even now, at 29, it happens occasionally. I don't share a bed with my husband, but he doesn't know why I don't want to, I'm too embarrassed to tell him — I'm sure he'd laugh at me if he knew. When I was a child my sisters used to tease me about it, and my mum used to tell the neighbours. I was sure everyone looked down on me because of it. I'm still very sensitive about the subject, and if it comes up in conversation with other mothers I never admit I used to wet the bed as a child, let alone tell them it still happens. Mothers still seem to think that a child who wets the bed does it deliberately — it's not true. I longed to stop, but I just couldn't help it. You can't control it — it happens when you're asleep.'

*Carole*

'Both my children, aged six and four, wet the bed at least twice a night. I'm finding it harder to cope with as they get older — I've asked everyone about it — health visitors, doctors, school nurse — and I've had a lot of conflicting advice. No one is willing to give any proper help or professional treatment until a child reaches seven.'

*Nicky*

'Alexander's wetting causes a bit of stress and strain. I'm relaxed about it, really, but his older brother makes sneering references occasionally to his friends — such as "this room stinks" because we used to keep a potty in it.'

*Lillian*

'He's very embarrassed about the fact that he still wets the bed.'

*Georgina*

'My son's five and he wets the bed every night. I'm at my wits' end. I've been told by the G.P. and the specialist that the problem's normal. They say it's not seriously treated until the age of seven. All I can see is another two years of hell.'

*Peggy*

One of the most graphic accounts of the feelings engendered by bed-wetting is found in playwright John Osborne's autobiography:
'For years I suffered the humiliation of being a fairly regular bed-wetter. I had not yet discovered that this was a common affliction and that the lone unfortunate bed-wetters themselves conspired unknowingly in their own isolation, each one intimidated into believing that he or she was a toad-like creature who made a swamp of beds in defiance of all that was decent.'[2]

Bed-wetting can add to a family's existing problems, and make them more difficult to solve. A social worker is quoted in one survey of the problem, describing the impact of bed-wetting in a family she is involved with '....there is bedding to be washed...and nightclothes and all this takes a lot of hot water, which is expensive. The family's supplementary benefit does not easily cover the cost involved and they are ashamed to ask for a grant for new mattresses...'[3]

Another social worker talked about eight-year-old David's mother:

'She is disabled...and finds it sometimes impossible to keep up with the washing. She has no effective spin-dryer or wringer and cannot hang her washing out unless she is able to keep her eyes on it all the time (it might get stolen). The electric oven usually provides the most effective method of drying washing.'[4]

After the age of three or so, we expect children to be making some sort of progress towards being dry at night as well as in the day. Many do — though in the London survey quoted above[5] 55 per cent of boys and 40 per cent of girls were still wet at night at three. Gradually the numbers wetting become smaller, though by school age it is still *very* common. Parents by this stage may have decided to take some steps to reduce the likelihood of wet beds but this isn't really active 'training'. Whether or not these steps have any effect on actual bladder behaviour is questionable. Most surveys indicate that something like 10–15 per cent of five-year-olds wet their beds. It's difficult to get precise figures as researchers differ in their definitions of how often is 'often' or 'regularly' but here are a few recent examples. In a study of children on the Isle of Wight[6], 13.4 per cent of boys and 13.9 per cent of girls 'sometimes' wet the bed. A study of 12000 children from all over the U.K., researched for the National Child Development Study, showed that 10.7 per cent of children between five and seven years of age wet the bed.[7] There seems to be no difference between boys and girls at the younger end of the age group, but as time goes on the difference becomes wider. The Isle of Wight survey showed that the proportion of boys wetting at seven was down to 6.7 per cent — but it was only 3.3 per cent of girls. The National Child Development Study showed that the proportion of bed-wetting children had dropped to 4.8 per cent at eleven.

Occasional bed-wetting is even more common — at the

age of five, 20 per cent of boys wet the bed at least once a month, and 21 per cent girls.[8] And when the parents of 1753 children aged between five and thirteen in California were questioned, 14 per cent reported at least one episode of enuresis in the preceding three months.[9]

It's a problem that has been regarded through the ages as a difficult one. An historical account[10] of different treatments describes things that make your hair stand on end. To quote Pliny the elder in the first century, 'the incontinence of urine in infants is checked by giving boiled mice in their food' and he also recommended wood lice and pig's urine. In the sixteenth century, the favourite solution was powdered claw of goat, and powdered hedgehog. The Victorians favoured nerve tonics, enemas, cold baths, hot baths, and a particularly horrendous sounding concoction of strychnine mixed with sheep fat, formed into a suppository and inserted several times daily into the rectum. Then they got enthusiastic about burning the urinary meatus (the opening of the urethra) with silver nitrate. To avoid the need for anaesthesia they put a few drops of cocaine directly into the urethra, though there's a documented case of a three-year-old (yes, three) who needed 12 separate shots of anaesthetic during the operation. Then they reckoned the removal of the tonsils and adenoids would do the trick. Various tight bandages were suggested, wrapped round the penis. There are two reported cases of the penis being cut away as a result of the bandages being too tight for too long.

A more liberal, less invasive approach was suggested in the 1920s — enuretic children should be taken away from school in case other children made fun of them. Instead, they should live carefree lives in the country, with plenty of fresh air and exercise.

As recently as the 1940s at least one American doctor was taking his young enuretic patients out into the crowded waiting-room and announcing their affliction to his captive audience — but I'm relieved to say this is unheard of now.

Not all doctors are confident about the way they deal with bed-wetting, however. A paediatrician has written admitting of a lack of satisfaction in his own attempts to help his patients and adds, 'a good many paediatricians would admit to similar reactions. They would be unwise to make their admissions known to the parents of these unfortunate children.'[11] This is unnecessarily gloomy an outlook, however. With the right approach, and treatment where necessary, bed-wetting can be helped — but sometimes the parents have to look hard for that help on behalf of the child, and to understand something of what's available themselves. As a specialist in this field has written, 'Many children have used various routines and treatments with disappointing results, because knowledge of the techniques and details of their practical use is nowhere near available enough to either parents or professionals.'[12].

There are two important truths that any parent worried about bed-wetting should remember: the first is that as your child grows up, he is less and less likely to persist in wetting the bed, and the second is that the majority of bed-wetters can be 'cured', given the right sort of help and guidance. These facts should be reassuring in themselves — no matter how maddening all that washing is, and how frustrating the situation is, it will (probably) stop.

One further truth you should never forget, too, is that *your child can't help it.* He is urinating in his sleep, and he has as much control over that as he has about the subjects of his dreams. Accepting that fact is important to your child, to your relationship with him, and to the outcome of any treatment he may undergo, as we'll see on page 103. And we'll also find out how you can get help, if you feel your child needs it (page 120).

## Types of bed-wetting and its causes.

Doctors normally divide enuresis into two categories, primary and secondary. Primary enuresis is bed-wetting occurring in a child who's never been dry at night, or not for any long period of time (definitions of a 'long' period of time vary — six months to a year is fairly typical, though). Secondary enuresis describes bed-wetting that has begun again in a child who has been successfully dry at night for a long time, (again, say six months to a year). It's usually accepted that secondary enuresis is a response to some stressful event in the child's life. Sometimes, however, the stress goes away or is coped with by the child, but the enuresis remains. Treatment for primary enuresis doesn't usually differ from treatment of secondary enuresis, though there may be special situations that could be dealt with, if the stress in the child's life remains, for example, and is somehow removable.

It's sometimes suggested[13] that adverse events occurring between the ages of say 2½ and 4, when the child would otherwise have become able to be dry all night, can interfere with the process and lead to bed-wetting. This is difficult to be sure about, as many happy and serene children from stable, loving families are bed-wetters (though the likelihood of bed-wetting is greater when there are family problems, see page 93). It's also likely, if we include things like the birth of a new sibling, starting playgroup, moving house, mum returning to work, death of a grandparent, a stay in hospital, that the majority of pre-schoolers experience some life-changing event. It could be that some children are more sensitive than others, of course, and it's known, after all, that stress can delay other areas of development, including day-time potty-training.

Bed-wetting certainly seems to run in families, which suggests there may be a genetic or inherited element, or perhaps a social or cultural influence on the child's development in this respect.

There's some evidence to indicate that children with a relatively small bladder capacity are more likely to wet the bed, and that this is also implicated in day-wetting, (see page 91). Children who sleep deeply may also wet the bed — several of the mothers included in my survey mentioned this as a presumed contributing factor — and failure to arouse oneself from this very deep sleep may well be a factor. A recent research round-up reckoned that the relationship between enuresis and sleep needs further investigating[14]. It's interesting to remember, in this context, that adult heavy drinkers are often bed-wetters, too, presumably because their sleep is so deep they don't wake up with the need to urinate.

## Treatment of bed-wetting

Many doctors are reluctant to consider dealing with the problem of bed-wetting until the child reaches the age of six or seven (see Nicky's and Peggy's stories on page 96). There are reasons for this, the main one being that about half the children wetting at five will have stopped by themselves by the age of seven. Letting nature, and the child's own development, take its course obviously pays off in 50 per cent or so of cases. Some of the aspects of treatment (such as the buzzer alarm on page 104) seem to work best when the child is old enough to co-operate, and there's certainly some justification for the idea that drawing a child's attention to his bedwetting by treating him for it may increase his anxiety, or cause anxiety before he's had a chance to grow out of it.

That said, mothers struggling with washing and their own feelings do need help. This may be given in a reassuring chat with the family doctor or health visitor, or by hearing other mothers admit to having the same problems and being able to benefit from a communal moan about them. Very practical ideas to cut down on the hard work and extra costs are on page 109.

### Star Charts

If your child's responsive and able to co-operate, you could try a star chart before the 'magic age' of seven. It worked with Maxine's son (page 62) for example, and in another part of her report Nicky says her elder child responded well to a star chart — though the success was short-lived and she relapsed afterwards. Basically, a star chart is made up of some sort of grid, with a space for each day — enough for at least a week. You may have a different grid to start each new week. For each night the child is dry you draw or stick a star in the appropriate space. You could give an extra special star — a gold one, perhaps — if the child is dry say three nights running, or after maybe seven stars not necessarily won on consecutive days.

This mild 'reward' system has much to recommend it. The child isn't punished for a wet night — all that happens is she doesn't get a star. She has a visible sign of any progress she makes and this seems to engender a real sense of achievement when success occurs.

You can be imaginative with a star chart. It doesn't have to be a chart, and it doesn't have to be stars. Some ideas I've seen or heard about include buying comic-book type stickers (available in newsagents) depicting a favourite character or perhaps animals and allowing the child to place them in an album; using a large, boldly-outlined picture of (say) a clown, and numbering different parts of him, '1' on his nose, '2' on his hat, '3' and '4' on each shoe and so on, which the child can colour in when he's dry. You can name each part with a day of the week, and start each new week with a new clown picture instead. You can use your imagination to work out what turns your child on.

Don't persist with the star chart, in whatever form you use it, if it's not having an effect. Leave it a while and try again later.

Incidentally, star charts can be used with advantages in other areas of behaviour. I had great success with one when I was trying to persuade my elder children to get dressed and downstairs in the morning without the usual fuss or distractions that risked us being late for school. They should only be used to focus on specific topics however. It's no use introducing them to improve your child's general behaviour, with a star for every day she's been 'good'. You need a definite goal — say a star for every day she hasn't bashed her little sister, or for every day she has tidied her room.

It's common to relapse after a star chart regime ceases, but there is no harm in starting one up again, if your child feels happy about it, after a gap. Do remember to be consistent about filling it in each morning — though if it becomes very effective, you may go through a few dry nights and forget to record them each time. That's all right — it shows the chart is coming to the end of its natural life.

## Going to the Doctor

If you do decide to seek further help for your child or your doctor feels it would be of some benefit then your own contribution and co-operation to the success of treatment will be greatly valued. In fact, a lot of the treatment will rely on you doing quite a large amount of the fundamentals at home between appointments. The doctor or other professional that you see will be offering back up and guidance while you do much of the work.

Treatment of bed-wetting is by no means standard wherever you go, and research goes on all the time to try and pinpoint the exact ingredients of success. However, most of the treatment nowadays does involve the elements of support for the child and family, practical encouragement (like a star chart) and the use of a buzzer alarm of some sort. There will probably be a purely medical aspect as well, at the beginning of treatment, because urine infections need to be checked and treated (see page 87) and rare abnormalities or disease, will have to be ruled out (the illness known as sickle cell disease or sickle cell anaemia for example can cause an excess of production of urine and hence enuresis).

It's possibly misleading to generalize, because each doctor may do some things in a different order and may not do some things at all. And it's as well to acknowledge at this point that although I'm referring to the doctor, this is a label of convenience. Your child may see a health visitor, a general practitioner (family doctor), a paediatrician (a children's specialist), a child psychiatrist, an 'ordinary' psychiatrist (both of whom are medical doctors), a clinical psychologist (who is not normally a doctor, or not of medicine anyway), an educational psychologist (not usually a doctor, either), the community physician (or a 'school doctor'), a social worker, a psychotherapist (not normally a doctor) — or any combination of these, not more than two or three at a time, however! It depends on who has the interest in giving help of this kind in your area and the job of carrying it on, (see page 120).

At your first appointment with the doctor, you'll be asked for some fairly full details of the extent of bed-wetting — how long it's been going on, how many times your child's wet per night, if she's ever dry or has ever been dry. You'll be asked about day-time bladder control, and about any history of bed-wetting in your family — both parents' sides. The doctor will want to know about anything else in the way of health problems or behaviour difficulties that are causing you concern, and how your child is progressing in all other respects, including her life at school, and he will ask you about your family life and what sort of housing you have. It may be that your child's school will be contacted for a report as well, and you'll be asked to keep a record of your child's bedwetting for a varying amount of time. You shouldn't find all this too daunting, as the doctor will have met this problem many times before. It's not uncommon for children to stop wetting during the record taking period, possibly because the doctor may continue to see them, giving support and encouragement, or because they may have been about to grow out of the wetting anyway[15]. It's not hard to conclude, however, that the good response in these cases may be a result of reassurance that someone is taking their problem seriously without overreacting to it. Children who become dry with these 'simple support measures' as one doctor calls them, rarely relapse, so the outlook is very good for them[16].

At later stages in the treatment, the doctor may suggest or give you a star chart of some sort for your child. If there is evidence that a more specialized form of therapy is needed for any behaviour problems, then your child might be referred for this, if the doctor doesn't feel capable of dealing with it, or prefers to keep treatment for enuresis separate. There may be other people who are informed of the treatment and of progress if they are not actually involved in it, such as the health visitor and possibly the school and the social services. You should be informed, however, if at any time this is the case. Social worker and health visitor support may be helpful if you need to apply to the DHSS for help with laundry costs, for example.

**Buzzer Alarms**
At some point the doctor may suggest the use of a buzzer

alarm to help your child's bed-wetting. Other names for this include the enuresis alarm, the bell and pad, a bleeper, or a bed-wetting alarm. There are a number of models on the market (see pages 111 and 140 for suppliers) but you'll probably have to use the one the doctor favours, or which the health authority supplies him with, at least at first.

Normally, the alarm is made up of either one or two pads connected via a lead to an alarm unit. The pad or pads are placed on the bottom sheet of the bed and then another sheet is placed on the top (with two pads you make a sandwich of sheet and pads). It's usually easiest to make the top sheet a draw sheet (an old cot or pram sheet is excellent). When your child goes to bed, he should lie on the bit of the bed where the pad is, having switched the alarm on. As soon as the pad is wet, salts in the urine complete an electrical circuit and the alarm goes off, by bleeping, buzzing, ringing or whatever. In some models a light flashes, too. The noise only stops when the alarm is switched off. This is supposed to wake your child up, and he then goes to the lavatory to finish emptying his bladder.

The sheets are changed, the pad(s) washed and dried and replaced, and the bed is remade as before. (Another, more simple-to-use alarm is described on page 109). The alarm should be switched on again before your child goes back to bed. Over a period of time — sometimes weeks, sometimes months — your child will become better at waking up sooner, and the amount of urine passed before waking will decrease, or he will manage to stop wetting altogether, and sleep through without needing to go to the toilet.

The mechanism whereby this is learnt by the child is set up by the way the alarm startles him when it goes off. This actually causes the sphincter muscle to tighten and the urine stops flowing temporarily. When he wakes up he recognizes the 'full bladder feeling' and goes to the toilet. Eventually, this tightening of the sphincter and the waking up become linked together and they happen without any deliberate effort.

## How successful is the alarm?
The alarm is by no means a guaranteed cure for bed-wetting

but it gives good results if it's used properly. Short-term results look excellent — one estimate is that on average 75 per cent of children start to improve within a very short time[17], and other doctors have found even better results. Total failures in this short-term are sometimes the result of the alarm not being properly used. The instructions need careful following and your doctor should take the time and trouble to explain its use, and it's often better if your health visitor or someone else comes to your house and actually demonstrates it to you and your child.

However, it's in the long-term that you'll be most interested in the success or otherwise of the alarm, and it's here that things don't look quite so easy. Some researchers have found relapse rates — that is, the number of children who start to wet the bed again after they have stopped using the alarm — to be very high. The average relapse rate has been estimated at 41 per cent of the 'initial success' children[18]. In some of these cases, treatment with the alarm is started again. When this was done in one study[19] a further sizeable proportion of the children became dry in the long-term, and when the whole study was completed, the number of children who were 'cured', after a follow-up lasting two years which made sure the cure was permanent, was 63 per cent. This is comparable with a similarly organized study in Liverpool published in 1985 when 67 per cent of children who completed the treatment were cured in the long-term[20].

**Ways of increasing the success**
There are a number of ways to help make a successful outcome more likely — and these are where *you* can help.

'Overlearning' is one example. This is a process which works on the theory that if someone can manage to train their bladder to work well under abnormal circumstances, it will work brilliantly well under normal ones. The buzzer alarm is used after the child has drunk up to two pints of liquid before bedtime (quite the opposite to what parents often do, which is to restrict them anytime after four or five o'clock in the afternoon). This means the child is actually far more likely to need to pass water than normal, and he gets a lot of use, at least initially, out of his buzzer alarm. Initial results of overlearning indicated that it can really help prevent children relapsing into bed-wetting once the buzzer treatment is stopped[21], but these results haven't continued to be borne out quite so dramatically.[22] Nevertheless, this is something that is worth considering, though it would need support and full co-operation from you, the parent, to get that much fluid into your child and also to be prepared to get out of bed several times in the night (especially with a younger child) to supervise the procedures involved in switching off the alarm, changing the sheets and switching it on again.

Other ways you can help your child and increase her chances of success with the treatment include remaining supportive, calm and tolerant of her problem. And as one study noted, 'the treatment of wetting problems of children generally depends upon time and effort expended by parents'.[23].

There is a group of children who are less likely to be successful at stopping bed-wetting. This group includes children who are in the older age groups; children from families with difficult social or relationship problems; children who wet during the day as well as during the night, (who, some researchers feel, need to be regarded as having a different sort of problem than the night-wetting children[24]); children with behaviour disorders; and children whose parents are intolerant of the bed-wetting and who do not co-operate well with treatment, or who aren't interested in following a professionally-run treatment programme.

### Other treatment

Some doctors prescribe drugs that work on the central nervous system in an attempt to damp down bladder activity, but these drugs have unpleasant side-effects in some cases, as well as being of doubtful long-term benefit. Accidental over-dosing has been noted as a hazard, too[25].

Some doctors suggest attempts to increase the bladder's capacity to 'hang on' during the day, by giving the child practice in taking large amounts of fluid and then not going to the lavatory immediately. The waiting period is gradually extended — but although this does appear to train the bladder to increase its capacity, it doesn't appear to have a direct effect on bed-wetting[26].

### Bed-wetting and allergy

One of the mothers I heard from seemed to have found a definite link between bed-wetting and allergy.

In this case, a 10 year-old boy had always wet the bed, and seemed actually worse on the prescribed medicine. A friend suggested the pink colouring in the medicine might be responsible, and inspired by this, the mother made sure all foods with artificial colouring were excluded from his diet. The bed-wetting ceased — 'but he only has to have school beefburgers, which have colouring in them, and he wets that night'.

### Strengthening the bladder sphincter

This can be an effective contribution to teaching the sphincter to remain closed, even when the child is in a deep sleep. One clinical psychologist working in the Midlands asks her patients to exercise this 'doughnut muscle' every time they go to the toilet. Her instructions tell the child 'instead of letting the water out all at once, stop and start the flow of water. As soon as you start to wee, count to two and stop; then count to two and start again; count to two and stop and so on until you have finished. The muscle will become stronger very gradually, so remember to do the exercise every single time you go to the toilet.'[27] It's similar to the pelvic-floor exercise taught to mothers after childbirth.

### Intensive methods

Intensive methods have been tried with 'night training'[28] with reportedly good results. The method needs a lot of commitment on behalf of child, parent and therapist, but it seems to work if it's done correctly. It incorporates hourly wakenings on the first week of training, and lots of 'positive practice' — getting the child to run through, up to 20 times, a sequence of events: lying down, getting up and going to the loo and then back to bed again. Professionals reading this can find a concise account of the procedure by obtaining a copy of the article cited in note 14. If parents are keen to try the method themselves, then go ahead. It may not suit you to go through all the 'positive practice' (it sounds very boring!) and instead you could try a few nights of frequent wakings after giving your child lots to drink.

## Practical notes

Buzzer alarms are used most effectively by children of at least six or seven, and with the back up and guidance of an experienced person. However, if the help you need isn't available it's possible to buy an alarm yourself from specialist suppliers.[29] Small, discreet alarms are now very widely produced — the alarm itself is pinned to the clothing and the pad used with it is a small stick-on disposable worn inside a normal pair of pants. This is more acceptable to most children and their parents, as the other sorts of pads are best used without pyjama bottoms. Actual wetting of the bed may be avoided, too, which is another plus point.

In fact, protecting the bed and somehow reducing the wash-load is very important, particularly when you remember a calm attitude helps your child. It may be difficult to remain calm if you have a load of wet bedding to deal with every morning. Protective mattress covers are essential, and an easily washed duvet and bottom sheet is helpful (choose nylon or polyester as opposed to cotton or wincyette). You could then add a drawsheet, possibly of plastic, and then a comfortable, easily washed sheet on top of this.

The Disabled Living Foundation (see page 69) has a very helpful set of guidelines on coping with bed-wetting plus a list of suppliers of aids such as waterproof sheets — contact them for details. You can also buy non-plastic protective duvet covers and pillowcases[30], which are placed between the duvet and the normal outer cover, and between the pillow and its normal case. Larger branches of Boots the chemist also have information and supplies.

Do watch the smell of urine-soaked beds — it can 'hang' round a bedroom unless you remove the bedding as soon as possible (stick it in a polythene bag if you need to change the bed in the middle of the night). And remember that a bed-wetting child needs a bath, shower or very thorough wash every morning or else he will be treated horribly at school.

If you are receiving state benefits, and you find the washing and drying is adding greatly to your heating bills, and increasing wear and tear on clothing, you may be able to claim extra help in the form of Additional Requirements payments or other allowances. You should ask at your local Citizens Advice Bureau, DHSS office or Social Services about eligibility.

1. See page 104
2. John Osborne *A Better Class of Person* (Faber and Faber, 1981). Quoted in *Enuresis in Schoolchildren* a discussion document issued in 1982 by Family Service Units
3. *Enuresis in Schoolchildren* op.cit.
4. ibid.
5. Weir op.cit.
6. M. Rutter, W. Yule, P. Graham in *Clinics in Developmental Medicine Numbers 48–49* (Heinemann, 1973)
7. J. Essen, C. Peckham (1976) *Nocturnal Enuresis in Childhood* (Developmental Medicine and Child Neurology, 18, 577–589)
8. W.C. Oppel, P.A. Harber, R.V. Rider (1968) *Social, physiological and neurological factors associated with nocturnal enuresis* (Pediatrics, 42, 627–641)
9. B. Foxman, R. Burciaga Valdez, R.H. Brook (1986) *Childhood enuresis — prevalence, perceived impact and prescribed treatments* (Pediatrics, 77, 482–487)
10. For example, M.A. Salmon (1975) *An historical account of nocturnal enuresis and its treatment* (Proceedings of the Royal Society of Medicine, 68, 443–445)
11. James Hutchison *Practical Paediatric Problems* (Lloyd Luke Limited, 1980)
12. Roger Morgan (1981) *Childhood Incontinence* (Heinemann, 1981)
13. For example, Sylvia Dische (1978) *Childhood enuresis: a family problem* (The Practitioner 221, 323–330)
14. D.M. Doleys, J.J. Dolce (1982) *Toilet training and enuresis* (Pediatric Clinics of North America 29, 297–313)

15. S. Dische, W. Yule, J. Corbett, D. Hand (1983) *Childhood nocturnal enuresis: factors associated with outcome of treatment with an enuresis alarm* (Developmental Medicine and Child Neurology, 25, 67–80)
16. ibid.
17. D.M. Doleys (1977) *Behavioural treatments for nocturnal enuresis in children: a review of the recent literature* (Psychological Bulletin, 84, 30–54)
18. ibid.
19. Dische et al op.cit.
20. D.M. Fielding (1985) *Factors associated with drop-out, relapse and failure in the conditioning treatment of nocturnal enuresis* (Behavioural Psychotherapy, 13, 174–185)
21. G.C. Young, R.T.T. Morgan (1972, 1973) *Overlearning in the conditioning treatment of enuresis* and *Analysis of factors associated with the extinction of a conditioned reflex* (Behaviour Research and Therapy 10, 418–420; 11, 219–221)
22. P.D. Taylor, R.K. Turner (1975) *A clinical trial of continuous, intermittent and overlearning "bell and pad" treatments for enuresis* (Behaviour Research and Therapy, 13, 281–293)
23. D.M. Fielding op.cit,
24. For example, D.M. Fielding (1982) *An analysis of the behaviour of day and night wetting children: towards a model of micturition control* (Behaviour Research and Therapy, 20, 49–60)
25. Foxman et al op.cit.
26. D.M. Doleys *Enuresis* in Advances in Behavioural Medicine (Spectrum, 1980)
27. Acknowledgement to Jennifer Adams, West Birmingham Health Authority
28. N.H. Azrin, T.J. Sneed, R.M. Foxx (1974) *Dry-bed training: rapid elimination of childhood enuresis* (Behaviour Research and Therapy, 12, 147–156)
29. Suppliers include Nottingham Rehab, 17 Ludlow Hill Road, West Bridgford, Nottingham NG2 6HD; Eastleigh Enuresis Alarms, 70 Nursery Road, London N14 5QH
30. From Squires Protective Bedding, 30 Clarence Road, Chesterfield, Derbyshire S40 1LN

# 15.

# SOILING

Soiling — passing bowel movements somewhere other than the lavatory or potty after the child is expected to have been trained, to use its broadest definition — can be very upsetting. It happens during the day, it makes a child messy and smelly and it is an absolute no-no, socially speaking, in any child over the age of about three in our society. Dirty pants are certainly viewed even more unfavourably than wet ones, on the whole, and as the child gets older it becomes a source of much shame.

It's very possibly something that's commoner than surveys suggest, simply because of the reluctance of parents to disclose the problem. Two large surveys indicated that at the age of seven, 2.3 per cent of boys and 0.7 per cent of girls were regular soilers[1] and at the age of eleven, the proportion was 1.3 per cent of boys and 0.3 per cent of girls[2]. It's far more common in boys than girls, but for both sexes it disappears by the mid-teenage years except as a part of severe psychotic disorders.

Soiling in younger children — say under the age of four or so — is best dealt with by giving lots of love and attention and switching your focus away from your child's bowel habits (see page 130). It's actually quite common and whether it's a combination of a delay in the development of bowel control or a way of expressing anger and frustration, no one can be really sure. With patience, however, it's often grown out of. If it turns out that your young child is very constipated (see page 80) you should think about changing his diet and seeking your doctor's advice.

The term used by some therapists to describe the phenomenon of soiling in older children is encopresis, but

# SOILING

this is defined by some as only referring to children who pass fully-formed bowel motions in their pants or somewhere else. The majority of soilers inadvertently leak faecal matter between (usually infrequent) visits to the toilet, rather than fully opening their bowels away from the toilet. This makes parents think that the problem is actually diarrhoea, as the faecal matter is sometimes more or less liquid, and it seems to happen without the child knowing about it, which is rather suggestive of the urgency associated with diarrhoea.

However, the truth is that this sort of soiling is a direct result of constipation.

'My eight-year-old son Martin has always been prone to constipation, and from the age of four he began to soil his pants regularly. It still happens about twice a week, and he loses so much at times that I have to change his bedding as it can happen during the night.'

*Erica*

What happens is that the child does not empty his bowels (for a variety of reasons, as we'll see). The uneliminated faeces remain in the rectum and the lower bowel and become harder and dryer — in fact, like rocks. The bowel becomes swollen, and the tissue it's made of stretches and stretches to make room for the faeces. Eventually, the nerve fibres that would normally respond to this by sending messages to the brain to tell the child to go to the toilet, become so stretched they lose their ability to respond. So the child stops feeling the need to empty his bowels. But he's still eating and his body still needs to eliminate the waste. There's really no room left for any more faeces, so the waste matter seeps out in a liquid or semi-soiled form through the crevices between the 'rocks'. The child doesn't feel it coming out, and only discovers it on his pants, or like Erica's son, on the sheets. Truly severe, chronic constipation like this sometimes has a physical cause — poor diet, abnormality of the intestine — but it's far more often associated with a fear or dislike of opening the bowels. Once constipation starts it can become worse, as we saw earlier on, because it becomes painful to pass the stools. If the bowel is eventually evacuated — and in constipated children this may only happen every week or even more rarely — the motions can actually clog up the household's plumbing. Then the cycle of faecal retention — 'hanging on' — begins again, because the underlying factor hasn't gone away. In very bad cases the child hardly ever passes a normal motion, and the leaking ('diarrhoea by-pass' as it's sometimes called — see Annie's story on page 83) is a daily occurrence. Sometimes normal motions are passed for a little while — and then the problem comes back again.

The leaking can be anything from a smear just staining the underwear, or a great deal more than that at times.

It seems to be, from various studies of soiling children, that half of them have never really acquired normal control of the bowels, and the other half started to soil sometime after control was achieved.[3]

It's universally admitted that soiling is a very difficult problem to solve. It can take literally years, and as one doctor says, 'the physician, the parents and the child easily become disenchanted with one another'. The child really does need a lot of support — especially as the soiling can lead to bullying and ragging at school, feelings of negativism and a chronic lack of self-confidence, plus a perpetual fear that other people will discover his shameful secret. He cannot help his problem — it's beyond his conscious control. He needs sympathy and the promise of help.

Getting at the root causes of the problem is not easy. There may be many factors involved. These include harsh, over-aggressive potty-training; a nagging insistence on a regular bowel habit on the part of the parent; fears of the toilet (see pages 57 and 83); previous prolonged illness which affected the bowels (such as gastro-enteritis); a poor relationship with the mother and father; excessive use of laxatives or suppositories when the child has had constipation (real or imaginary) before; not allowing enough time on the toilet for defecation to complete itself; rushing out to school every morning and not making space for a visit to the lavatory; other social stresses with which the child finds it difficult to cope.

# SOILING

There's rarely any one single cause for this form of faecal retention, and it's likely that each child has a number of unconscious 'reasons' why he ends up so bunged-up that soiling is the result.

Sometimes, the problem may begin as a reaction to starting school, or starting at a new school. This isn't just because the situation presents new stresses to upset a sensitive child. It's often because of the school toilets. A child may come to school and discover there are no locks on the toilet door, or it's the place where the school bullies attack their victims, or perhaps there's hardly ever any toilet paper. There may be constant flooding from leaky cisterns, or the less-than-perfect hygiene of other children may make the toilets unpleasant to use. As I've heard my own children say more than once, 'our school loos really *stink*!' Under these circumstances it's easy to understand how a child may want to 'go' when he's at school, decide to put it off until he gets home, and then find the urge has gone by 4 o'clock. If this sequence continues every day he can be well and truly blocked after a while.

It's true to say that children who soil often have a problem with disturbed behaviour and they may come from unstable families. But this is by no means always the case. Most experts will deal with each case as individually as possible — 'it should never be assumed that a child with bowel incontinence is "emotionally disturbed".[4] It can happen of course that the soiling can lead to disturbed behaviour, as it's such a distressing symptom.

Professional help for encopretic children will be given mainly by doctors and therapists such as the ones listed on page 103 who may deal with enuresis. It's important for you and your child to *like* the doctor looking after you and to try to establish a good relationship — the length of time the treatment may take will mean you'll be seeing a lot of each other.

Your child will be given a physical examination, and true abnormalities of the intestine will be ruled out. The chances are he'll be discovered to be very constipated and the doctor's first move in the way of actual treatment will be to 'clean him out' with a prescription for laxatives (or maybe enemas or suppositories), the dosage and type given according to the degree of constipation.

Girls with encopresis may have a urinary infection, and this will be checked for at this time.

If there is an anal fissure (see page 84) the doctor will prescribe medication to soften the stools, and possibly anaesthetic ointment to relieve the pain when the motion is passed.

Some doctors favour admitting the child to hospital if the constipation is bad enough to warrant it, or if the child needs to be observed and it's difficult to reach a conclusion about the extent of the problem in any other way, or if the doctor doesn't reckon the parents will be very co-operative in seeing the treatment is actually given.

The doctor will also want a detailed history of the soiling, and an account of your child's toilet-training plus information about your family life. The toilet arrangements in your house or the child's school are important (and the doctor will want to know if there's any other obvious factor that's putting the child off going to the toilet). There'll be the chance for you to give information about past and present illnesses. It could be that your child suffers from recurrent tummy pains, for example. The doctor may be able to reassure you on this point, as frequent pains are often a direct result of infrequent bowel actions.[5]

The doctor who's experienced in helping encopretic children will want to make sure you will stop punishing your child for his soiling, and to try and do what one doctor calls 'demystification' of the whole subject by explaining exactly what has happened with his bowels and toileting. He'll want to reassure your child by convincing him that he's not so unusual, that (as the same doctor put it) 'other cool guys also have a messing problem'. Doctors on this side of the Atlantic might put it another way of course!

Over the period of treatment, the doctor may decide to ask you to make sure your child makes a regular point of visiting the toilet, such as after meals, and staying there for a few minutes or longer. Younger children might like a supply of colouring books and crayons to help them pass the time. A star chart might be valuable to keep up the interest — you'll award a star for every session on the toilet, whether anything is produced or not, at least at first. New toilet habits have to be learnt and forgotten bowel sensations remembered again. It may take time.

Your child will continue to have laxatives and/or stool softeners prescribed to help prevent any build-up of faeces, and between visits to the doctor, you the parent will be asked to keep a record of bowel actions and toilet visits (older children may be asked to do this themselves, if the doctor feels they are reliable).

There may be times when the doctor wants to see your child alone, and he may feel you as a family need support and back-up, as well as encouragement in maintaining the (possibly new) regime of no punishment for messy pants. You won't be expected to accept your child's non-co-operation with the treatment, however, and you will be 'allowed' to get annoyed if it helps to make sure your child takes his medicine and makes his scheduled visits to the toilet. Your child's diet may need some change too, to increase fibre content.

Commonly, treatment like this produces temporary success, and then the child relapses. But eventually, it produces a permanent cure in over 90 per cent of cases.[6]

There's some evidence to suggest that children who need laxatives for a long time have forgotten, or have never learnt, to co-ordinate their muscles in order to defecate properly.[7] Researchers compared a group of encopretic children with a group of non-encopretic children. In what sounds like a rather uncomfortable experiment, the two groups were asked to pass a water filled balloon, and by means of electrodes, internal pressure and muscle activity were monitored and compared. The encopretic group seemed to 'strain' incorrectly and inefficiently — leading to speculation that some sort of abnormality in the musculature of the pelvic-floor was involved in encopresis. However, this inability to defecate properly could just as easily be the *result* of encopresis, and more research needs to be done in this area. It could be also that over-anxious potty-training may affect the muscle action — hurrying the child or forcing the child to sit for ages on the pot. Trying to 'hold back' while simultaneously defecating because, unconsciously or consciously, the child doesn't want to defecate, could affect it, too, and then it could become a habit that's hard to unlearn.

There are some practical measures you can take to help minimize your child's unhappiness and embarrassment about his problem — would it be possible for instance to arrange for a permanent 'excused' note from games and PE at school? This might mean informing the school of the situation and engaging their compliance in some sort of 'cover-up' to let other children think your child's got a bad back or flat feet or something similarly vague. Let the school know if the toilets there are truly awful — in the case of fear of bullying in the toilets increased supervision is essential. For younger children in an infants school or younger juniors it may be possible to actively engage the help of auxilliary staff in monitoring toilet visits, and keeping a record of 'accidents'.

A small group of children start to soil without underlying constipation.

'Since my husband and I divorced — very traumatically — a year ago, my six-year-old son has soiled his pants almost every day. He's not constipated, he doesn't like doing it, but he says he doesn't know why it happens.'
*Marjorie*

'Samuel is five and every time something adverse happens, he soils his pants. I'm by no means the world's most patient person, and I'm often in tears with rage and frustration at it all.'
*Linda*

This is always a difficult problem to cope with, and when it happens regularly over a period of time it's a sign of underlying stress and unhappiness. It's much rarer in the older age groups, and eventually children do somehow grow out of the tendency — but at great cost, in many cases, in terms of family relationships and self-confidence of the child. Special help is needed to pinpoint the difficulties in the child's life and to help him and his family overcome them.

Occasionally, children aged four and five soil because toilet-training has been absolutely non-existent — nobody's bothered to encourage the child to use the toilet — or the training has just gone so wrong for some reason that progress has been minimal. A health visitor or a social worker can step in here once it's certain that lack of training or poor training is the main culprit, and give advice on getting the child trained.

Children beyond the toddler stage who regularly and deliberately smear faeces are also crying out for help. I'm not referring to the toddler left on her own for a few minutes with a dirty nappy that's come unstuck or unpinned, or the one who opens her bowels in the garden on a sunny day when she's got no clothes on, both of whom are liable to play with their faeces out of sheer novelty and curiosity (I'm sure most parents have a horror story to tell!). If that happens, by the way, don't throw a fit of disgust and shock. Simply tell your child that we don't do that sort of thing, thank you very much. It's the older child, pre-school and older, who does this who is expressing some deep aggression and frustration — and it needs professional therapy to find out why.

1. M. Bellman (1966) *Studies on encopresis* (Acta Pediatrica Scandinavica, Supplement 170)
2. M. Rutter et al op.cit. note 6, p.110
3. For example, Bellman op.cit.
4. M.D. Levine (1982) *Encopresis: its potentiation, evaluation and alleviation* (Pediatric Clinics of North America 29, 315–330)
5. N.V. Freeman (1978) *Faecal soiling and constipation in children* (The Practitioner 221, 333–337)
6. ibid.
7. V.A. Loening-Fauke, B.M. Cruickshank (1986) *Abnormal defecation dynamics in chronically constipated children with encopresis* (Journal of Pediatrics, 108, 562–566)

# 16.

# WHERE TO FIND HELP

In the United Kingdom, your first port of call when you have a problem related in some way to health is your family doctor. Through him, or her, you can have access to the wider range of specialist knowledge in child guidance clinics, paediatric or psychiatric outpatients, at the hospital, counselling services and so on. Your family doctor should know, or should be able to find out, if there are any special clinics locally, run for children with wetting and soiling problems. These are relatively few and far between, but if you find one near you, a referral to it is a way of getting help from people who have experience in dealing with these problems, and just as important, an interest in this area. Your health visitor, the school doctor or the educational psychologist may make a referral in some areas — it can depend on local protocol. Some paediatricians for example, only accept referrals from the family doctor. Child guidance clinics will be well-used to having referrals from other sources, and some will even accept referrals from parents themselves.

Your Community Health Council (in Scotland the Local Health Council) may be able to help you by letting you know what's available in your area, or you could try the local education department or the social services for information too.

Your **family doctor** may well be more than capable of dealing with the problem, without referring you on, especially if he's a sympathetic person who relates well to children. In a recent report[1] 95 per cent of G.P.s surveyed reckoned to deal with the problem of enuresis themselves, for example. I don't suppose all of them have 100 per cent success rates, however, and if you feel your family doctor hasn't solved the problem, or doesn't show enough interest, then do ask to be referred to a specialist or to a clinic. Don't struggle on, the way so many of us are tempted to do, saying 'even the doctor couldn't help him'. Tell the doctor the problem's still there, otherwise he'll think he's managed a 'cure', and you can ask for further help.

**Health visitors** are especially helpful with younger children who aren't at the stage of having a major problem. Your health visitor is able to talk over the way you're managing toilet-training, and her experience with young families and her knowledge of you and your circumstances, may be better than the G.P.'s. You can ask for a home visit from your health visitor, or you can visit her at the clinic. Some health centres have special 'toddler sessions' which could be very suitable.

Try not to feel guilty if you need to go outside the family to help your child. Don't feel angry with your child for having put you in a situation where you're admitting 'I can't cope.' It's not *his* fault, and it's not *your* fault. None of us is perfect, but the majority of us do our best according to our circumstances and the emotional and psychological baggage we're obliged to bring with us into parenthood. You, too, will have done your best, and if you love your child, showing him that love will be the best support you can give him. You may think you've done things 'all wrong' — but that may have been what you thought was right at the time. Starting off on an optimistic new footing with treatment that may lead to a cure, that you can work on together with your child, will help you cope with any feelings of guilt or anger, overcome them and then finally forget them.

1. *Children and Prevention in General Practice* — a report for the Regional Advisory Group on health promotion and preventive medicine, West Midlands Health Services, 1984.

# QUESTIONS AND ANSWERS

**They've started bed-wetting**
Q. *Both my sons were very quick at potty-training and they were out of nappies well before the age of three. They're now aged five and four, and since I remarried last year they have both wet the bed almost every night. I've been very easy-going about it, but my husband's reaction is quite different. He doesn't actually punish them, but the situation does cause a lot of upset between us because of the difference in our attitudes. Is there anything I can do?*

A. I'm sure you know children often need to show distress by regressing in their toilet habits, and that includes bed-wetting. Your own calm reaction is the right one — this is something that's outside your children's conscious control and getting cross is not only unproductive, but actually rather unkind. Allow yourself and your husband to acknowledge the 'nuisance factor' of extra washing by all means, but without showing direct irritation towards your children. Let your children have the chance to talk about their feelings. Maybe they're worried that their new daddy will go away — or even that you will go away.

Your husband probably sees the bed-wetting as a reflection of the way the children feel about him, and he's understandably sensitive to anything that indicates everything's less than perfect. But for the sake of your children, you both need to be consistent in your approach. Support your children, let them know you're sure they will soon go back to having dry nights, and that if the problem continues you'll get special help (via the doctor or health visitor) for them.

## Dirty every morning

Q. *My 3½ year old son is still in nappies at night, and he's dirty almost every morning. What can I do about this?*

A. It's highly unlikely your son is opening his bowels in his sleep, and he's probably doing it as soon as he wakes in the morning. If this isn't too uncivilized an hour for you, you could try going in to him at this time with the potty, or actually get him out of bed and take him to the toilet. He will be able to understand if you explain to him that he should shout to you if he needs to open his bowels — or at this age you could be encouraging independence anyway by suggesting he get up and go by himself. Of course, many three year olds still need their bottoms wiping, so you'll have to accept getting out of bed for this. Don't be too concerned about the situation though — he's likely to grow out of it soon.

## He likes nappies

Q. *I've asked 2½ year-old Nicholas if he'd like to use the potty several times but he's always refused. Do you think he might be wanting to be like his baby sister in some way, preferring to cling on to babyhood by remaining in nappies? I know I should wait for him to ask to use the potty but I'd like to hurry him along somehow.*

A. At 2½ your little boy may just be slightly slower to train than others of his age — or it could be that he just likes being in nappies and hasn't seen any point in not needing them. It's a bit soon to speculate on whether he has any deep-seated longing to be a baby or dread of growing up. It's actually more likely that going without nappies isn't really a positive prospect — so why should he bother? You could be a little less laid-back about potty-training if you wanted to. Hanging back waiting for him to ask could mean a long wait if he has yet to fully understand what the potty and toilet are for and how pleased you'd be if he used them. Borrow a friend's son to show your own son how big it is to wear pants instead of nappies. You can let him see that he's different from his little sister because he's your big boy, and special in his own right because of that. All of this

## Bed-wetting at 12

Q. *My son is 12 and he has more-or-less always wet the bed. We did have some help from the doctor a few years ago but after six months or so he went back to wetting. He's terribly embarrassed about it, and he's made me promise not to go to the doctor again and tell him the problem is still there. What can we do? He'd love to go away to Scout camp this summer, but it's just not possible while the wetting continues.*

A. Relapse after successful treatment for bed-wetting isn't uncommon (see page 104) but in the long term the outlook for bed-wetters is reasonably good. This means that with the right treatment your son's bed-wetting should be cured — and many bed-wetters stop at puberty anyway, which your son will reach within the next couple of years or so. Tell your son that there's hope for him, and tell him also that you will keep your promise not to tell anyone about his problem. Instead he's old enough to take responsibility himself. Don't change his sheets for him, or his pyjamas. Leave clean sheets and pyjamas where he can get them himself, and get him to deal with the practical side of bed-wetting without your help. He is also old enough to go and see the doctor himself, and to describe the situation without you being there. If a referral to a specialist or to a clinic is made, the doctor or therapist may wish to see you too, but there's no reason why the initial contact can't be made with your son. Tell your son that getting help now may cure him in a matter of weeks — soon enough for Scout camp.

## She just forgets

Q. *My daughter's very bright and intelligent but she still has occasional accidents at the age of 3¼. She often says by way of explanation 'Mummy, I just forgot'. Is this possible? Shouldn't it be automatic by now?*

A. Many three-year-olds have accidents, even if they're otherwise almost independent regarding the toilet. Yet it certainly is possible for a child to 'forget' — most especially when she's absorbed in something else. Somehow the brain hasn't yet learned to be insistent enough in reminding the child that the 'full' feeling means the child will have to go soon or she'll have an accident. Young children haven't yet developed the feeling of social strictness that would allow fear of shame and embarrassment to prevent urination away from the lavatory except under the most extreme circumstances. The result is that the bladder opens — to the child's genuine surprise.

### Is it diarrhoea?

Q. *Is it possible for a breastfed baby to have diarrhoea? My baby is six weeks old, and fully breastfed, and his stools seem very loose. Occasionally, he has a stool which is green in colour, and I usually reckon on having at least four or five dirty nappies a day. My friend who's also breastfeeding has two separate nappy buckets — one for 'wet only' and one for 'dirty'. There'd be no point in my doing that, as the 'wet' bucket would hardly get any contributions.*

A. Both your babies sound perfectly normal — neither of those very different bowel habits are a sign of ill-health. Loose stools are normal in a breastfed — sometimes they may be no more than a smear or a stain on the nappy. Breastfed babies' stools are actually less offensive than those of bottle-fed babies; though they may certainly be more copious at times, they smell quite reasonable! The odd green stool in a healthy baby is insignificant — it's merely a sign of what is sometimes called 'intestinal hurry', when the gut has been a little more active in digesting than usual. Diarrhoea in a *fully* breastfed baby is virtually unknown: breast milk gives a great deal of protection against it, and there are also less opportunities for diarrhoea — causing bugs to enter the system — anyway.

## Maternal pressure

Q. *My mother keeps making pointed remarks about potty-training — she thinks I'm leaving it far too late. But to me Zoe is too young at 18 months to try. How can I avoid feeling irritated at my mother's pressure?*

A. Irritation is a reasonably justified reaction! Potty-training practices have changed down the generations and no one can say which is definitely right, but you are 'in charge' and you should do what you feel is right for you and your daughter. It's interesting to note that the 'modern way' of relatively late training goes back to what our grandmothers and great grandmothers did. According to American paediatricians[1] the prevailing attitude towards toilet-training was one of permissiveness until the 1930s. Then leniency changed to rigidity: 'The use of very strict and structured schedules was the rule, and the techniques were frequently co-ercive in nature.'[2] This was also the era when rigid feeding schedules were recommended, on fairly spurious physiological grounds as we now know. The New Zealand psychiatrist Truby King had one of the first truly best selling babycare books in the Western world, and mothers followed his advice to fit their babies into a routine for practically everything.

The pendulum hasn't taken that long to swing back, however, and we regard inflexibility and early training as just not for us. Why don't you have a frank word with your mother? Point out that the evidence showing early trained children reach true toileting independence much earlier just doesn't exist, and that you'd prefer to avoid the hard work of active training before your child's likely to be ready. Then ask her to let the matter rest with you.

## Fussy eater

Q. *My daughter's five and very fussy about her food. She hardly eats any fruit and vegetables, and this results in severe bouts of constipation. How can I improve her diet — and therefore her bowel actions?*

A. It's important never to force-feed a child, but there are ways to gradually increase the range of foods a child will eat. It's very sensible to think of ways you can do this, because, as you've found, lack of fibre in the diet does indeed lead to constipation. At the age of five your daughter will be able to understand a simplified explanation of the way her body and digestive system work, and you may be able to get her to co-operate as a result. After all, she won't enjoy being constipated, and if you can convince her that changing her eating will help, you may find her more willing. Wholegrain cereals and pulses are good sources of fibre, and you can experiment by trying out some sorts that are a little out-of-the-ordinary. You can buy whole oats, whole rye and millet from health and wholefood shops, along with pulses you might not have tried before. Will your daughter eat vegetable soup? You can make this with extra quantities of beans and other pulses, and perhaps with a handful of whole grain barley. Vegetables are sometimes more acceptable raw, cut into sticks like the French do and served as 'crudités' to dip into mayonnaise or other sauces. Only the very best veg should be used like this — fresh, crisp and crunchy, rather than old and soft. Make sure the cereal she has in the morning is made with wholegrains — Weetabix, Farmhouse Bran, Shreddies, are all popular with children — porridge is another suggestion.

She may like dried fruit if she's not keen on fresh fruit — dried prunes and dried apricots are fairly widely available. Healthy snack foods such as 'Tropical Mix' which you can buy by the quarter or half pound in some supermarkets has a lot of fibre-full bits and pieces in it. You should also check your daughter's fluid intake (see page 82).

### Is he slow?

Q. *Oliver is 26 months old, and he's really slow at being toilet-trained. I've been trying to get the message over for three months now — he just wets his pants more often than not. I know he could do it if he wanted to, because there are odd occasions when he tells me in advance. He makes such a lot of extra mess and washing that I can't help getting angry with him.*

A. Getting angry with Oliver will delay his progress, and if you don't feel you can cope with the situation calmly, then it might be better just to put him back into nappies for a couple of months before trying again. Elsewhere in this book you'll see that 26 months isn't late in being clean and dry, and as Oliver can tell you some of the time when he wants the potty he's obviously on the way to being trained. He can't really help his frequent accidents — at just turned two you're asking quite a lot of someone who may not be quite ready physically or emotionally to co-operate all the time with your ideals!

### Early birth

Q. *My son was born eight weeks prematurely and weighed only 3½ pounds. After that difficult start in life, though, he recovered well, and has no health problems at all. At the age of two years nine months however, he's still not toilet-trained. Could this early birth have anything to do with this?*

A. Possibly. At least one research study[3] found that babies weighing less than 2500 grams at birth — that's 5½ pounds — were later than babies of average or above average weight at being dry day and night.

### Sore bottom

Q. *Since my daughter's been out of nappies in the daytime, she seems to have developed a tendency to a sore bottom. It's as if her skin has stopped being used to a wet nappy, and the night nappy she still wears seems to be the cause of her soreness.*

A. It's certainly probable that your daughter's night nappy will be aggravating her sore bottom, whatever the original cause of it. Could it be that with only the one nappy in every 24 hours you aren't paying quite so much attention to rinsing the nappies out after washing or sterilizing? Most parents wash the nappies in a machine, but you may be doing it by hand as you have so few at a time — and there may be traces of nappy sterilizing powder or detergent left in them. Stubborn rashes on the bottom, the sort that won't get any better after home treatment with a baby cream, vaseline or zinc and castor oil, need to be looked at by a doctor. It could be for instance, that your daughter's soreness has some underlying fungal infection like thrush. In the meantime, make sure you wash your daughter's bottom thoroughly every morning with soap and hot water, and that she's then properly dried before putting any cream on.

**Dry before clean**

Q. *I know most children learn to control their bowels before their bladders, but my daughter Melanie is quite the opposite. She became dry in the day about six weeks ago, but she seems to be taking ages to be reliable about her bowel motions. She knows when she's done it, and comes to me to have her pants changed. She's just over two.*

A. It's very early days. Don't worry about it and don't allow Melanie to worry about it, and you will almost certainly find she manages to achieve bowel control. It might be helpful to make a note of when a bowel motion is likely to happen — Melanie may open her bowels at more or less the same time each day, and she may give definite signs that one is on the way. (Some children become a bit fidgety or restless, for instance.) You can then remind her about the potty, or quickly take her there or to the toilet.

**Wet pants at $4\frac{1}{2}$**

Q. *Jo is 4½ and she still wets her pants. I honestly don't think it's stress or anxiety and the doctor has ruled out urinary tract infection or any other abnormality. She just isn't 'trained' properly. I've tried everything, bribery, threats, smacking, shouting, extra cuddles, you name it, I've tried it. I am at my wits' end.*

A. Calm down! Yes, it must be frustrating to feel you've gone through every possible trick in the book with no success, but you and Jo have got yourselves caught up in a vicious circle which needs to be broken. Tell Jo that you're truly sorry toilet-training has made you both so cross with each other, but that now she's a big girl you feel you can work together happily to achieve dryness. Choose a good moment, when you're not angry or irritated with her, for this little heart-to-heart. Tell her you know that she's a clever, big girl deep down, and she's clever and big enough to *want* to be dry like all her friends. Then you could consider having an intensive day with the toilet (not the potty) as described on page 29, or else have a slightly less intensive weekend, when reminders to go to the toilet are given very frequently. Reward Jo with a small treat every time you see her pants are still dry (check for this every half-hour or so) and also for when she uses the toilet correctly. Keep the atmosphere happy and keep up the praise. Forget about the two or three years of non-productive training and pretend you are starting from scratch. If this doesn't help, then see your health visitor or family doctor.

**I get so angry with her**
Q. *I'm finding it very hard to cope with my daughter's soiling. She's 2½ and I've been told my feelings are important in the 'cure' — if I fail to be roused to anger she'll be more likely to co-operate. But it really 'gets' to me. Any ideas?*
A. Remember that *you* are the mature, thinking person in this relationship — and as an adult it really should be possible to cope with your reactions sensibly. If you can do this, you will see results. You know from this experience that anger and frustration haven't helped, so logic should convince you to try it the other way. When your daughter soils, just clean her up and ask her to use the potty or toilet next time. To quote from one excellent book on the problems parents have with their children[4]: 'Make sure you don't become entirely centred on her bottom in your contact with her, but make special times during the day when you can play together and have a pleasurable time.' Your daughter needs to know she can get your attention other than by soiling so it's worth really making these 'special times' a priority. Even 20 minutes a day of your undivided attention, as long as it is consistent and reliable, will make a real difference.

## Occasional wet beds

Q. *My four-year-old daughter has been out of nappies at night for a year and she usually gets out of bed if she needs a wee and goes to the toilet without disturbing anyone. However, we still have the occasional wet bed — sometimes a couple of nights running. Is this normal?*

A. Yes, it's very common. Short-lived lapses in control like this are still a normal part of life for many young children. They're sometimes associated with excitement at a forthcoming event, and excitement after a particularly hilarious outing or birthday party — and often children who are ill wet the bed. Holidays and weekends away from home may mean a setback, especially if your child's not entirely sure where the toilet is, or is afraid to get up in the dark in a strange house.

## Funny little ways!

Q. *My daughter hates the thought of her bowel motion splashing water up from the toilet — and although she's now seven, she still floats loo paper on top of the water so 'it' can have a papery, rather than a watery, landing. It used to irritate me a bit, but now I accept it.*

A. You're absolutely right to accept it. Lots of children have idiosyncratic toilet procedures and as long as they're not anti-social in any way, or difficult for the child and the rest of the family to live with, then there's no harm in an otherwise healthy and well-balanced child. If you had the nerve to ask, I bet you'd find some adults have peculiarities, as well! I know a very sensible, highly paid executive who admitted he always operated the flush handle on the loo with his elbow, even at home, reasoning (not totally without cause) that the handle is the germiest place in the bathroom, because people touch it after using the loo but before washing their hands. And many of us would (almost) rather die than use a public loo that was not up to perfect cleanliness standard.

## He needs a nappy on

Q. *My son is 26 months, and he has excellent bladder and*

*bowel control. However, he always wants me to put a nappy on him when he needs to open his bowels. So far I've complied with this request but I don't know if I'm doing the right thing.*

A. You'd be surprised how common this is. There's something about passing a bowel motion that some children dislike. Perhaps it's feeling that it's part of their body that's 'falling off' (see page 135), and perhaps they don't like pushing it out into the empty space of a toilet or potty. The nappy gives them a feeling of security. I think you're right to go along with this, and you're almost certain to find your son simply grows out of the dislike of the potty and toilet within a very short time. You can let him know in the meantime that you're sure he'll be able to manage to use the potty instead soon — don't get annoyed with him but don't let him think you find his nappy reliance totally acceptable, either. Do be careful not to put pressure on him though — he's still very young, and doing very well to be in control of his bowels and bladder.

### Circumcision and wetting

Q. *When Jonathon was just three, he was circumcised because his foreskin was too tight and he was getting infection after infection. He was more or less fully trained before his operation but since then he's started wetting again, during the day and the night.*

A. You'll need to go back to your doctor and ask his advice as it's certainly possible that Jonathon has developed a urine infection. You'll need to consider the possibilities that the stay in hospital has affected his feelings about urinating, and about his penis. It's not always easy to explain about hospitals and operations to very small children and they can get some funny ideas about what has happened. It might help if Jonathon can somehow see another circumcised penis on another boy, and if he's given a chance to talk about what he feels about urinating and about the different appearance of his penis. As a parent, you'll have the chance to bring these aspects into the conversation in a reasonably natural and unforced way.

Think, too, about whether simply the experience of being in hospital and separated from familiar surroundings, even for a short time, can have upset him. If the problem doesn't resolve itself, ask your G.P. for professional help.

**"Giggle Micturition"**
Q. *My son is twelve, and he has a problem he's almost too embarrassed to discuss with me. He empties his bladder when laughing — I mean completely empties it. He's had no problems with bed-wetting, and he's never wet his pants since being a toddler.*
A. This is a rare problem — though it's probably commoner than you might think, because like your son people are ashamed to admit to it. It's termed 'giggle micturition' in the medical literature, and it's defined as 'complete, involuntary, unstoppable emptying of the bladder on laughter'[5] by two Leeds paediatricians reporting on a pair of cases they had studied. Your son should be helped with the right treatment — this might mean medication for a short period of time, together with encouragement and sympathy. Ask your doctor for referral to a paediatrician or to a clinic dealing with enuresis.

**He won't stand up**
Q. *My son is three, and although he's been using the toilet for a good few months he won't stand up to pee — he prefers to sit down. I'm a single parent so he hasn't got a dad to show him.*
A. Please don't worry about this. Many boys take a while to get used to standing up when urinating, but they will, eventually. When your child starts nursery school or playgroup he will see what other boys are doing and just want to copy. If he doesn't at first, then, again, be patient. Just remind him as casually as you can that big boys and men do it standing up — if you can borrow a friendly male friend or relative for a quick demonstration it could help. Don't make your son anxious about it, though.

## Bottom wiping

Q. *When should a child learn to wipe his or her own bottom? We've got two children, aged three and four, and the favourite cry in our house is 'someone come and wipe my bottom please'.*

A. Lots of the mothers I heard from highlighted this aspect of independence in toileting as the last one to be reached, and there were plenty of four-year-olds (and older) who preferred mum to do it. It's a skill that has to be taught, and practised, and of course many mothers do it for their children for longer than they thought they would, because the child isn't terribly efficient at it.

You should aim to have your children independently wiping by school age, or you will be *persona non grata* on parents' night! Think of that poor reception class teacher — imagine if she had to wipe up to 30 bottoms a day. Teach girls to wipe from front to back to avoid the risk of infections and make sure both sexes remember to wash and dry their hands afterwards, and flush the loo, too.

## Bribery and corruption department

Q. *Do bribes and rewards have any part to play in toilet-training? Can they do more harm than good?*

A. I suppose some parents start off saying they'll never bribe their children to do anything and then actually stick to that principle through thick and thin. What saints!

I'm of the opinion that *used sensibly* a bit of bribery never did anyone any harm. The posh psychological term is 'positive reinforcement', meaning that if one sort of behaviour leads to something nice happening, your child is more likely to repeat the behaviour that led up to the nice thing. It's common sense, really, and it does work in many cases. However, lots of people potty-train without bribing or rewarding — except by giving praise or verbal encouragement — so it's by no means a vital piece of your strategy. You know your child, if you think he's really ready to learn about bowel and bladder control and capable of co-operating given the will to do so, an intelligent use of bribes (not threats, bribes!) is fine. Many of the mothers I heard from used this form of very tangible encouragement — one child had a small square of chocolate for every performance, another was allowed to tear his own toilet paper off, another (see page 58) was given a cup of her favourite drink. The trick is to keep it low-key and don't for goodness sake let your child up the stakes. The tale is told in one text-book of the child who used to ask his mother 'what will you give me if I use the pot today?' (for a bowel motion).[6] I don't think threats are a good idea, mainly because they introduce unpleasantness into a process which should be kept enjoyable, and because they can so easily escalate into positively unkind intolerant behaviour on the parent's part. This will hinder training, not help it.

### The buzzer's too loud

Q. *Please help. The buzzer alarm we have bought for my son is helpful, but it wakes the whole house up as well. We have two other children and we don't like the thought of their sleep being disturbed every night.*

A. You could try the sort of 'silent awakener' alarm that vibrates the pillow instead of making a noise.[7] This is just as effective, and may be even better than the buzzer alarm for children who sleep so deeply they don't hear the buzzer. There is also a smaller model that is worn by the child which vibrates against the body.[8]

### Fear of the stool

Q. *In one of my baby books, it says that young children can get very frightened of passing a stool because they feel it's part of them that's disappearing. Is this true?*

A. This idea seems quite popular in America, for some reason! Dr Benjamin Spock, doctor and author of one of the world's best selling baby books ever, advises parents to empty the potty into the toilet and flush after the child is out of the room, in case the child develops a fear that bits of him will get swirled away, too.[9] And Dr T Berry Brazelton, another American, talks about anxiety as a result of the toddler 'giving up' his bowel movement to the toilet and allowing it to go down the drain.[10] According to him it's a common phenomenon.

It's possible that there's some truth in this, although as with everything to do with toddlers who can't actually articulate many of their deepest feelings, it has to be speculative. It may exist as a factor in the problem older children sometimes have of retaining their faeces. Personally though, I think that Spock and Brazelton, distinguished as they are, exaggerate, at least as far as non-American children are concerned. Taking avoiding action by only emptying the potty when the child can't see would be inconvenient in most households and impossible with a curious toddler around. Anyway, if he doesn't see where it goes, how does he know for sure what happens to it? I really don't think it's important enough to worry about unless your child actually develops what seems to be a fear, when it may give you an insight into what's bothering him.

### He insists on the potty

Q. *My son is absolutely terrified of the toilet — I don't know why. The result is that at 3½ he still uses the potty, and only under the most extreme pressure and need will he use the lavatory in anyone else's house, and then only for a wee. He would never do a poo anywhere but in his own potty. We feel he's far too old to be insisting on having a potty, but we don't know how to change him.*

A. Something may have happened to frighten your son when he was using the toilet one day. Perhaps he slipped off the seat, or maybe the lid came down suddenly and gave him a fright. Other children may have scared him with tales of 'monsters living in the loo' — the chances are he's forgotten what put him off in the first place, and that's why he can't tell you what his objections are. All that remains is the fear, which will be genuine and difficult to overcome. Try bearing with him through this stage. He'll soon realize that other children use the loo and he is unlikely to want to be different. If the situation is upsetting you, though, tell yourself to keep it in perspective. It doesn't really matter, does it, if he uses the potty? If times goes on and you feel he needs a little encouragement, then you can offer to stay with him when he's in the loo or leave the bathroom door open — and maybe use a bit of low-key bribery for every time he uses it. You could certainly insist, even at this stage, that he uses the potty in the bathroom rather than anywhere else in the house. You could also consider a child's toilet seat if you don't already use one.

## He's started masturbating

Q. *Since I've been potty-training, my son has become very interested in playing with his penis — usually when he sits on the potty, waiting to 'do' something, but during other times as well.*

A. I'm sure you can guess what your reaction should *not* be. Slapping his hand and saying 'filthy boy' or words to that effect is not appropriate to what is after all a natural activity. Almost everyone — man, woman, girl, boy — masturbates in some way at some time, and it's perfectly understandable that being able to get at his penis, now it's not layered in nappy, is gratifying to your son. However, the fact remains that it's not socially acceptable in public, and your son will eventually have to appreciate that. It may reassure you to know that mothers of girls come up against the same issue, too, and severe disapproval and punishment is just as inappropriate.

If it bothers you, reduce his sitting time on the pot (there's little to be gained from letting him stay there for ages, unless you feel it's *really* helping with the training) and keep his attention from wandering by talking or reading to him. While he's young, gently distract him, perhaps by giving him something to hold for you if he starts masturbating (he'll need something that takes two hands to hold). As he gets older, if it's still a 'problem', explain that although you understand that playing with his penis is comforting and sometimes especially pleasurable, it's something that 'big people' do when they're on their own, in private. The same explanation goes for girls who 'play with themselves'. Persistent masturbation in both sexes despite parental guidance as to the 'where' and the 'when' may need professional help — but this isn't the case with a toddler.

## Constipation

Q. *Ever since he was a toddler, my five-year-old son has had a tendency to constipation. In fact, he's been on laxatives prescribed by the doctor more or less continuously for three years. Every time I try to take him off his regular dose he gets 'bunged up'. Should I worry?*

A. Many children do seem to take laxatives for long periods of times, with the same reaction as your son if the medication is stopped. However, it isn't ideal, as it's preventing the bowel from developing its own rhythm and action. Children can become dependent on regular laxatives, and this leads to what I have heard described as a 'flabby' bowel. It should be possible to gradually reduce the dose, however, and to temporarily substitute different, gentler-acting medicine if necessary. The sorts of medicines generally prescribed for constipation fall into three groups: firstly, the purgatives, which directly encourage the bowel to move; secondly, the preparations which increase the faecal mass by bulking it out; and thirdly, the stool softeners, which make the stool more comfortable to pass. Generally-speaking, purgatives should not be prescribed for a long period unless there's an over-riding reason (for instance, the child is receiving treatment for encopresis, see page 115). The important thing, however, is to discuss your worries with your doctor, and not to expect an instant return to normal.

## Stains on the settee

Q. *My daughter had rather a bad accident on the settee at my sister-in-law's house — in fact, she soiled her pants, which leaked all over the beige fabric — the mark's still there, and I'd love to be able to get rid of it and salve my conscience.*

A. Stains like these are usually best dealt with immediately, but even so, it's still well worth trying to tackle it.

As a guide, carpets and upholstery with urine or faeces on them need to be sponged with plenty of cool water, and then dried with a clean cloth. Then you can apply a diluted carpet or upholstery shampoo — repeated applications may be necessary on a large stain. If this treatment doesn't get rid of it, try a solution of white vinegar in water and gently sponge the stain. You do need to be careful to avoid a water mark with some fabrics when the sponging has dried — always work from the centre of the stain out, and don't get the fabric too wet. A hair dryer can be used to dry the fabric, which will speed up the drying process considerably. On washable fabrics, biological washing powder and liquids should get rid of stains without any problem.

### Toilet-training and hang-ups

Q. *Is it true that the way you potty-train your child can have an effect on his or her sexuality later on?*

A. This is another of those guilt inducing strictures that could really worry you if you let it! Toilet-training is only one small part of childhood, one small part of the many years of interaction you will have with your child. Psychoanalytic theory posits links between training and subsequent personality, and that does include, it's true, adult sexuality. If potty-training is carried out in a cruel and punitive way, then it seems to me that much else that goes on between a parent and child will be cruel and punitive. It will be this whole atmosphere, and the lack of love in the relationship, that is likely to affect the child in the long-term. Fortunately, writers and experts who say things like 'special care must be taken not to infect the child with disgust towards his body and its products. Harsh and hasty measures may make the child feel that his body and all of its functions are something to dread rather than to enjoy'[11] are less likely to pontificate to mothers these days. Most parents realize that 'harsh and hasty measures' are inappropriate because they're unkind and ineffective — we don't have to be forced into a state of nervousness in case we mess up our child's sex life by introducing the potty at the wrong moment! And I do think it's sad that parents are still sometimes made to feel that the effect of mistakes they made in the past can't be altered in any way, or that they can be held to blame for anything and everything that goes wrong with the child's adult relationships. Take heart from what columnist Katherine Whitehorn quotes as 'Foulkes Law of Random Results: that in child rearing, as in management or war, the results are only randomly related to the efforts of the people in charge.'[12] In other words, your children may make a mess of their lives, but don't blame yourselves. And I would add, don't blame potty-training!

1. D.M. Doleys, J.J. Dolce *Toilet training and enuresis* (Pediatric clinics of North America 1982, 29, 297–313)
2. ibid.
3. W.C. Oppel, P.A. Harper, R.V. Rider (Pediatrics 1968, 42, 614–626)
4. Jo Douglas and Naomi Richman *Coping with young children* (Penguin, 1984)
5. J.T. Brocklebank, S.R. Meadow (1981) *Cure of giggle micturition* (Archives of Diseases in Childhood, 56, 232–234)
6. R.S. Illingworth *The Normal Child* (Churchill Livingstone, 1983)
7. See manufacturers' addresses, page 111
8. Write for details to Aremco, Grove House, Lenham, Kent ME17 2PX. Telephone 0622 858502
9. Dr Benjamin Spock *Baby and Child Care* (Star Books, 1976 edition)
10. Dr T. Berry Brazelton *Toddlers and Parents* (Pelican, 1979)
11. Haim G. Ginnott *Between Parent and Child* (Pan, 1969)
12. Katherine Whitehorn in *The Observer*, November 16, 1986

# INDEX

'accidents' (*see also* wetting and soiling)
  parental attitudes to 48–51
  practical measures 52
  removing stains 138–9
  at school 90, 115, 118
aeroplane journeys 57
age, and toilet
  training 19–22
allergy
  and bed-wetting 108
  and diarrhoea 86
anal fissure 84–5
anal sphincter muscle 14

Balinitis 88
bed-wetting 94–111
  adult 94–5, 100
  and allergy 108
  and heredity 100
  practical measures 109–110
  statistics 97–8
  treatment 101–110
  types of 99–101
bladder 12–13
bleeding from anus 85
bottle-fed babies
  diarrhoea in 86
  stools of 15
bottom
  sore 92, 128–9
  wiping 87, 134

bowel motions (*see* stools)
bowels 14
breastfed babies
  diarrhoea in 86, 125
  stools of 15
buzzer alarms 95, 104–107, 109, 135

car journeys 56–7
'child's initiative'
  approach 26–8
circumcision 132
clothes, covenience while
  training 46
constipation 80–84
  and soiling 113–9
co-ordination, and readiness
  for training 35–6

DHSS, help with laundry
  costs 104, 110
delays in achieving
  control 73–79
diarrhoea 85–7, 125
diarrhoea by-pass 113–4
diet and constipation 81–2, 127
Disabled Living
  Foundation 69, 109
disposable nappy pads 54–5
doctor 84, 88, 92, 98–9, 103–4, 107, 115–7, 120–1

drugs to control
  urination 92, 107

'early approach' to
  training 24–26
emotional readiness for
  training 36–7
encopresis *see* soiling
enuresis *see* bed-wetting

fibre 81, 127
food intolerance 86
foreskin 88, 132

general principles 43–7
giggle micturition 133

handicapped children 66-9
  mentally 67
  physically 68-9
health visitors 121
Hirschsprung's disease 88
holidays 56–7
hypospadias 88

increasing fluid intake 40
'intensive' approach 28–30

kidneys 12

laxatives 84, 137–8
'lifting' at night 62–3

masturbation 137
mattress covers 63–4
meconium 14
medical help 103, 120

nephrons 12
night-time control 60–64

outings, and visits to the
  toilet 53–6

parental anxiety, and training
  delays 75–7
pelvic floor muscles 91
physical abnormalities 88
physical handicap 68–9
physical readiness for
  training 35
potty
  different types 43–4
  how to clean 44
primary enuresis 99
protective covers for
  bedding 109
psychiatric disturbance 92
public toilets 55

readiness for training 35–7
reflex actions 26
restricting fluids in
  evening 63
rewards 102, 135

school
  and 'accidents' 90, 115, 118
  toilets 115, 118
secondary enuresis 99–100
seepage of urine 92–3
sex differences, and
  training 12, 78–9
sexuality, effect of toilet
  training on 139
shops, finding a toilet
  in 55–6
sickle cell anaemia 103
soiling 112–9
  professional help 115–7
sore bottom 92, 128–9
sphincter muscle 12, 108
'standard British dead-slow-
  and-stop' approach 30–33
star charts 62, 101–2
statistics on wetting and

soiling 21, 77–8, 97–8, 112
stools
  composition 14
  fear of 135–6
  frequency 15
suggested programme of training 39–42

toilet, fear of 83, 136–7
toilet seat 41–2, 44–5
toilet step 45
trainer pants 45–6
travelling 56–7
twins 65–6

unexpected success 58–9
unfamiliar toilets 57

ureters 12
urgency 14
urinary tract infections 87–8
urination, basics of 12–3
urodynamic biofeedback 91

verbal readiness for training 36
vomiting 86

wetting
  day-time 90–93
  night-time *see* bed-wetting
wetting dolls 29
wetness indicators on nappy 35
words to use 46–7

**Other recommended reading...**

# THE KIDS WORK OUT GUIDE FOR PARENTS

## Dr John Pearce

Being a parent isn't an easy job—but help is at hand!

THE KIDS WORK OUT GUIDE FOR PARENTS is a comprehensive source of advice, giving solutions to everyday problems, easy-to-remember guidelines and answers to all the 'Yes, but ... What if ...?' questions you ever wanted to ask.

Such topics as bedtime problems, temper tantrums, jealousy, keeping safe, and many more are dealt with thoroughly in this lively, easy-to-understand guide by television child expert Dr John Pearce.

So, if you've got kids—whether they are newborn babies or lively 12 year olds—this book is for you!